Lorraine Maynard

1' Reactive Depression:
Resulting ~~existence incident~~ from a
particular incident.

Situation + reaction = illness

Tonic } 2 Stages of
Clonic } convulsions

Psychology in the Classroom
Author - Rudolph Dreikurs, M.D.
Published by Harper.
~~Suffer~~ Professor of Psychiatry @ Chicago
Med. School - Teacher.
Author: The Challenge of Marriage
        The Challenge of ~~Parenthood~~.

Types of restraints
1) mechanical -
2) manual -
3) Chemical -

PSYCHIATRY FOR NURSES

PSYCHIATRY FOR NURSES

PSYCHIATRY FOR NURSES

BY

LOUIS J. KARNOSH, B.S., Sc.D., M.D.

Associate Clinical Professor of Nervous Diseases, School of Medicine,
Western Reserve University; Director of Neuropsychiatry, City
Hospital, Cleveland; Consulting Neuropsychiatrist,
Cleveland Clinic

AND

EDITH B. GAGE, R.N.

Formerly Supervisor, Neuropsychiatric Division,
City Hospital, Cleveland

IN COLLABORATION WITH

DOROTHY MERENESS, A.B., M.N., R.N.

Instructor of Psychiatric Nursing, Neuropsychiatric Division,
City Hospital, Cleveland

Illustrated

SECOND EDITION

ST. LOUIS
THE C. V. MOSBY COMPANY
1944

COPYRIGHT, 1940, 1944, BY THE C. V. MOSBY COMPANY

(All rights reserved)

Reprinted, 1944

Printed in the
United States of America

Press of
The C. V. Mosby Company
St. Louis

To

FRANCES PAYNE BOLTON
Patron of the nursing arts
and tireless champion of
higher standards in
nursing education

PREFACE TO SECOND EDITION

Textbooks age very rapidly; their usefulness diminishes quickly and, like other necessary devices, they require periodic repair. This revision is justified not only because "Psychiatry for Nurses" has met with a gratifying reception, but because within the last three years, research has added steadily to our knowledge of the diagnosis and treatment of mental afflictions. The war and its repercussions upon the individual and upon society in general have revealed new problems and new methods of study of human behavior.

Only a few items can be cited of the many new increments of psychiatry. Such, for example, are the interesting revelations made through the technique of electroencephalography, the Rorschach and other tests in studying personality and the emphasis on body-mind relationship presented by the new psychosomatic medicine. In the field of therapy one can point to the remarkably simple and effective electric shock and to the newer therapeutic agents in treating epilepsy. The list of references has naturally been amplified and again emphasis has been focused upon the nursing features of each type of psychosis.

The authors express their obligations and gratitude to willing workers who made the task of revision a pleasant one. Particular mention is made of Drs. Edward Zucker and H. A. Lipson for editorial and advisory aid and to Mr. Frank Gaynor for the photographic contributions.

Louis J. Karnosh

Cleveland, Ohio

3

PREFACE TO FIRST EDITION

A textbook for students who are to be introduced to a new subject should contain the pith of that subject and very little more. The modern curriculum in a nursing school makes furious demands upon the mental capacities of the student. The rapid succession of "specialty courses" with their welter of new terms and their special techniques is particularly formidable to the beginner.

The specialist by the very nature of his calling is likely to be hyperenthusiastic in his desire to present many exquisite phases of his subject, and his temptation is to write a text that is cumbersome, that is technically too heavy for the beginner, and that is likely to frighten rather than to stimulate the student.

Some of the principles of psychiatry are a radical departure from those of orthodox medical practice. The proper introduction to this subject should be one which has a regard for this difference and should therefore emphasize the basic elements of psychiatry in as concrete and practical a manner as possible.

This textbook has been written with an eye to the peculiar needs of the nursing school of today, in which the student is required to familiarize herself quickly with the symptoms, terminology, and treatment of the more common psychoses as well as to recognize—perhaps for the first time—the importance of dealing with the whole personality of the sick person, no matter what the particular illness may be.

Emphasis on the various mental ailments presented in this text is in direct proportion to their frequency and their importance from the standpoint of therapy and nursing care. Hence the so-called biogenic disorders

4

such as manic-depressive psychoses, involutional psychoses, schizophrenia, paranoid states, and the psychoneuroses assume the more prominent portions in the text, and the new shock therapies applicable to some of these disturbances are given appropriate consideration.

Case histories enliven the text to present more clearly the specific features of each disease entity and to point out to the student nurse how significant is the life history of the psychotic person in understanding the manifold factors which come into play when personality is in distress. This broad concept of the disease process expresses the viewpoint of what is often termed the "American School of Psychiatry"—a point of view which not only makes for a better understanding of the mentally ill person but inculcates in the nurse a more hopeful and constructive attitude toward the patient.

It is hoped that the simple manner in which the subject is handled will inspire the nurse to look into the many ramifications which psychiatry offers, such as mental hygiene, vocational guidance, and administrative and nursing work with children, adolescents, and delinquents.

Only a few references to other texts are included. While this may be a departure from normal custom, it is argued that each instructor prefers her own favorite list. Moreover, contemporary knowledge and research in psychiatry is so rapidly expanding in all directions that any list of references included would become rapidly obsolete.

The requirements laid down by the National League of Nursing Education have been kept in mind during the construction of the text so far as the writers were capable of doing so.

Acknowledgment of greatly appreciated assistance is hereby expressed to the co-workers, both physicians and nurses, at the Psychiatric Division of Cleveland City Hospital, wherein the necessary experience and material for the book was obtained. Particularly grateful are the writers to Miss Opal McCray, who prepared the photographs which enhance the text no little degree, and to Dr. Roger F. Scherb, and Miss Mabel L. Leavitt, who assisted ably in coordination of the clinical data. Sincere appreciation is expressed for the inspiration and encouragement afforded by the publishers and their representatives.

Louis J. Karnosh
Edith B. Gage

Cleveland, Ohio

INTRODUCTION

In spite of the publicity given to mental illness and to psychiatric institutions in recent years, the general feeling still persists that nervous and mental maladies are uncanny and mystifying phenomena and that the nursing of those troubled with such disorders is a complicated and hazardous occupation. Many nurses who are about to enter training in a psychiatric hospital do so with vague fear and dread. As in everything else, this insecurity is due to a fear of the unknown. As this unknown sphere becomes familiar through experience gained by reading, by lectures, and by contact with the patient, confidence and poise replace doubt and misgiving. Very soon the nurse finds herself intrigued by the many phases and problems of psychiatry and even looks forward to emergencies which will test her capabilities. Many shy nurses, uncertain of their potentialities, have discovered their own real worth on the psychiatric wards.

Nursing mentally ill patients is a challenge to the intelligent, imaginative nurse. Imagination tempered with good common sense is a necessary requisite for persons dealing with those who are victims of mental and nervous disorders. Through this quality the nurse can sense in varying degrees the internal experiences of the patient. By understanding what lies behind the manifest symptoms of the trouble, she may more readily and adequately assist her charges as well as find the work itself less of a drudgery. The nurse finds her work interesting only in direct proportion to her knowledge of the ailment of her patient.

No two psychiatric patients are ever alike in personality, character, and display of symptomatology; hence by its very nature psychiatric nursing should never prove boresome or monotonous. The unfolding of the life history of a mental patient is a drama which should stimulate not only curiosity but a desire to broaden one's knowledge of human nature.

A nurse who is successful in caring for the mentally ill is by virtue of this ability equipped with certain qualities which will make her useful as a guide and advisor in many of the common psychological problems which confront the normal individual in the workaday world. The experience obtained on the psychiatric wards will benefit the nurse in all fields of medicine as it will facilitate handling and establishing rapport with many types of patient. Last, and by no means the least, she will develop that hallmark of culture—a tolerant attitude toward human frailty and an inexhaustible store of patience with all individuals with exaggerated traits of personality.

CONTENTS

10 CONTENTS

12 CONTENTS

ILLUSTRATIONS

14

PSYCHIATRY FOR NURSES

PSYCHIATRY FOR NURSES

PSYCHIATRY FOR NURSES

CHAPTER I

HISTORICAL REVIEW OF PSYCHIATRY

In his slow development through the ages primitive man gradually acquired a sense of compassion for his fellow-creatures; he then began to recognize mental disorders and to make attempts at treating them. In the light of modern knowledge these attempts were undeniably crude and meaningless.

From the study of contemporary primitive peoples and their attitude toward the mentally ill, it can be safely inferred that after certain tribal rites failed to effect a cure, the victim of mental disease in the dim past was disposed of by the simple expedient of being abandoned to shift for himself and to die quickly of starvation in a barren waste or to be devoured by animals in the wilderness. That some prehistoric peoples had, however, developed a high degree of knowledge about the brain and its functions is the conclusion of anthropologists who have studied the remains of several civilizations both in the new and the old world. Excavations have revealed skeletons that clearly bear evidences of successful trepanning of the skull which the subjects survived by several years. It is assumed that such operations were done to relieve headache and probably mental derangement and that even some knowledge of asepsis may have existed in those remote days.

In recorded ancient history such as that of the Eastern Mediterranean civilizations there are references to mental disorders. Thus, an Egyptian papyrus of 1500 B.C. contains a discourse on old age and says of it that "the heart grows heavy and remembers not yesterday." In later Egyptian civilization, particularly during the Alexandrian era, medicine developed a high status; sanatoria known as the temples of Saturn were operated for the care of those who were mentally afflicted. The Old Testament records authentic cases of mental illness, of which King Saul is a famous example.

The Golden Age of Greece was noted for its humane regard for the sick. The Greek physicians were poor anatomists because they deified the human body and dared not dissect it, but they were astute observers and excellent clinicians. Hippocrates (460-357? B.C.), the greatest of the old Greek physicians, knew well the symptoms of melancholia and regarded epilepsy not as the "sacred disease," but insisted that "it has a natural cause from which it originates like other afflictions." The Greeks used as hospitals temples which had an abundance of fresh air, pure water, and sunshine. These temples of Aesculapius "as often as they had patients, such as were unhinged, did make use of nothing so much for the cure of them as symphony and sweet harmony of voices." Theatricals, riding, walking, and listening to the sound of a waterfall were all recommended as methods to divert the melancholic. With this amazingly humane attitude, there were, however, instances where the treatment was not always free of its vicious aspects, for even in the best of the Greek temples, starving, chains, and flogging were advocated because with these it was believed that, when those who refused food began to eat, frequently the memory was also refreshed thereby.

There is a surprising paucity of data about the Roman era in reference to mental disease. Galen, who was actually a Greek, but practiced in Rome, based his treatment on the teachings of his Greek predecessors. Other physicians of the Roman era treated mental illness by bleeding, purging and with sulphur baths.

With the collapse of Greek and Roman civilization, along with other cultural accretions, medicine suffered an almost complete eclipse. The treatment of mental illness was left to priests and every sort of superstitious belief flourished. The insane were flogged, fettered, scourged, and starved in the belief that the devils which possessed them could be driven out by these means.

A few bright spots in this tragic picture were some monasteries or shrines where this technique of "exorcising" the evil spirit was performed by the gentle laying on of hands instead of the whip. Members of the nobility, self-appointed esthetes, and holy men of varying degrees of sincerity practiced this art, which at least had the fact to recommend it that it was not physically cruel.

Out of this tradition and belief in the "holy" or "royal touch" arose several great shrines, of which the one at Gheel in Belgium is most famous. The legend behind the beginnings of this colony is worth the telling. Somewhere in the dim past there lived a king in Ireland who was married to a most beautiful character and who sired an equally beautiful daughter. The good queen developed a fatal illness, and at her deathbed the daughter dedicated herself to a life of purity and service to the poor and the mentally bereft. The widowed king was beside himself with grief and announced to his subjects that he must at once be assuaged of sorrow by marrying the woman in his kingdom who most resembled the dead queen. No such paragon was found. But the devil came and whispered to the king that there was such a woman— his own daughter. The devil spurred the king to propose marriage to the girl, but she was appropriately outraged by this incestuous overture and fled across the English

Channel to Belgium. There the king overtook her and with Satan at his elbow, slew the girl and her faithful attendants. In the night the angels came, recapitated the body and concealed it in the forest near the village of Gheel. Years later five lunatics chained together spent the night with their keepers at a small wayside shrine near this Belgian village. Overnight all the victims recovered. Here indeed must be the place where the dead girl, reincarnated as St. Dymphna, was buried, and here was the sacred spot where her cures of the insane are effected. In the fifteenth century pilgrimages to Gheel from every part of the civilized world were organized for the mentally sick. Many of the pilgrims remained in Gheel to live with the inhabitants of the locality and in the passing years it became the natural thing to accept them into the homes and thus the first "colony" was formed and for that matter the only one which has been consistently successful. It continues to exist to the present day. Some 1,500 certified patients live in private homes, work with the inhabitants and suffer no particular restriction of freedom, except to refrain from visiting public places and from the use of alcohol and to report regularly to the supervising psychiatrist. In spite of the success of the Gheel colony and its great humanizing value, most attempts at duplicating it elsewhere have been complete or partial failures.

Although the treatment of the mentally ill in the Middle Ages had nothing much to recommend it, the period which followed was in some respects a great deal worse. When the church and the monastery gave up the care of the insane, it was gradually taken over by the so-called almshouse, the contract house and the secular asylum. The more violent patients gravitated to jails and dungeons. In the sixteenth century, Henry VIII officially dedicated Bethlem Hospital in London as a lunatic asylum. It soon became the notorious "Bedlam" whose hideous practices were immortalized by Hogarth, the famous cartoonist; whose keepers were allowed to exhibit the most boisterous of the patients for two pence a look and whose more harmless inmates were forced to seek charity on the streets of London as the "Bedlam beggars" of Shakespeare's *King Lear.*

In those dark days of psychiatry society was interested in its own self-security, not in the welfare of the insane. The almshouses were a combination of jail and asylum, and within their walls petty criminals and the insane were herded indiscriminately. In the seventeenth and eighteenth centuries the dungeons of Paris were the only places where the violently insane could be committed. Drastic purgings and bleedings were the favorite therapeutic procedures of the day and "mad-shirts" and the whip were applied religiously by the cell-keepers.

Superstition about mental disease took a horrible turn in the seventeenth century. God and Satan were still engaged in a ceaseless battle for possession of one's soul. The year after the "Mayflower" sailed into Plymouth Harbor, Burton published his classic work, entitled *Anatomy of Melancholy,* wherein he stated that "witches and magicians can cure and cause most diseases." To seek out and liquidate witches became a sacred religious duty. Twenty thousand persons were said to have been burned in Scotland alone during the seventeenth century. Small wonder that Cotton Mather precipitated the witch mania in Salem, for he was merely subscribing to the dogma of the day.

The political and social reformations in France toward the end of the eighteenth century permeated into the hospitals and jails of Paris. In 1792, Pinel, a young physician, was given permission by the Revolutionary Commune to liberate the miserable inmates of two of the largest hospitals, some of whom had been in chains for twenty years. Had his experiment proved a failure, he might well have lost his head by the guillotine. Fortunately he was right, for by his act he had proved conclusively the fallacy of inhuman treatment of the insane. The reforms instituted by Pinel were continued by his pupil, Esquirol, who founded no less than ten asylums and was the first regular teacher of psychiatry. The Quakers under the Brothers Tuke had at this time established the York Retreat and effected the same epoch-making reforms in England.

In America under the guidance of the ubiquitous Benjamin Franklin, the Pennsylvania Hospital was completed in 1756, where the insane were still relegated to the cellar but there at least they were assured clean bedding and warm rooms. Benjamin Rush, a prime humanitarian and the "father of American psychiatry," entered upon his duties at the Pennsylvania Hospital in 1783. Subscribing in part to the lunar theory of insanity, inventing an inhuman restraining device called the tranquillizer, but at the same time insisting on more humane treatment of the mentally afflicted, he stands as a prominent transitional figure between the old era and the new.

Most of the states were still without special institutions for the mentally ill in the first quarter of the nineteenth century. The poorhouse or almshouse was still popular, but it invariably became a catchall for all types of offenders, and the mentally ill received the brunt of its manifold evils. Most shocking to modern concepts was the placing of the poor and the mildly demented on the auction block, where those with the strongest backs and the weakest minds were sold to the highest bidder, the returns from the sale being assigned to the township treasury.

About 1830 a vigorous movement having for its object the erection of suitable state hospitals spread simultaneously through several states. The excellent results obtained by a private institution such as the Hartford Retreat, which was founded a few years before, probably served as an object lesson. Horace Mann took an enthusiastic interest in the plight of the insane, and the advantages of a state hospital system were publicized to promote construction of such institutions.

However, it remained for an asthenic, forty-year-old schoolteacher to expose to a torpid public the sins of the poorhouse. From that day in 1841 when Dorothea Lynde Dix described the hoarfrost on the walls of the cells of the East Somerville jail in Massachusetts to the day when she retreated into one of the very hospitals she was instrumental in creating, she effected reforms which shook the world. She so aroused the public conscience that millions of dollars were raised to build suitable hospitals and twenty states responded directly to her appeals. She played an important part in the founding of St. Elizabeth's Hospital in Washington, directed the opening of two large institutions in the maritime provinces of Canada, completely reformed the asylum system in Scotland and in several other foreign countries and rounded out a most amazing career by organizing the nursing forces of the northern armies during the Civil War. A resolution presented by the United States Congress in 1901 characterized her as "among the noblest examples of humanity in all history."

By the middle of the nineteenth century, the asylum, "the big house on the hill," became a familiar landmark in every state capital, ensconced in its landscaped park and topped by high turrets and senseless cupolas. In it mentally afflicted men and women lived and enjoyed a modicum of comfort and freedom from abuse. But to the general public it had a fortresslike appearance, and its occupants were a strange and foreboding lot. From this smug isolation the psychiatrist made no attempt to teach the man in the street anything to ease his fear and horror of mental disease. As a matter of fact, he could not impart much information, for he had little to give. While such matters as management, housing, and feeding of mental patients were slowly attaining decent humanitarian standards, as late as 1840 there was no clear classification of mental disorders and a German teacher, Doctor Heinroth, was still advancing the theory that insanity and sin were identical. Not until 1845 when Griesinger published the first authentic textbook on mental disease was the position of psychiatry in relation to other medical sciences clearly defined.

Formal research into the cause and nature of nervous and mental disease gained impetus under the inspiration of Jean Charcot, the great French neurologist whose clinics attracted students from every country in the world. Toward the end of the nineteenth century much new knowledge was derived from the microscopic study of the brain and the introduction of laboratory methods. The development of out-patient departments for psychiatric cases dates back to 1885 when persons suffering with incipient disease were treated at the Pennsylvania Hospital and a few months later at Warren in the same state.

The emphasis on prevention and recognition of early stages of mental illness was not made until the turn of the present century, when Clifford Beers entered upon the scene. Having spent several years in various mental institutions as a patient, he emerged in 1907 to write his famous book, *A Mind That Found Itself*. Being of a vivid, colorful temperament, he had unlimited enthusiasm which he directed in founding the National Committee for Mental Hygiene. Under the momentum of his aggressive leadership, the movement became worldwide and now has ramifications in the form of child guidance, prison psychiatry, vocational guidance and other practical activities, which concern the normal human being as much as they do the abnormal.

Coincidentally with the hygiene program came the astounding contributions of Sigmund Freud, which revolutionalized the orthodox concepts of mind, opened it by a new technique for exploration and brought psychiatry as a living subject to the attention of every intelligent man and woman. Psychiatry, at last, left its flying buttresses and ramparts and participated in everyday, human activity.

The last two decades are characterized by successful attacks on mental disorders by means of special physical remedies, even though psychoanalytic medicine still enjoys a huge following. Outstanding is the introduction of malaria and other types of fever therapy in 1917 by Wagner-Jauregg, which is now indispensable in treating neurosyphilis and chorea; the prolonged sleep treatment in agitated mental states with sodium amytal; the remarkable effects of vitamin principles on delirious and exhaustive states, such as alcoholism, pellagra and polyneuritis; and more recently the amazing and unique shock methods of treating schizophrenia with insulin as introduced by Sakel and the gratifying experiences in the treatment of mental depressions by the convulsion-producing drug known as metrazol, and by electric shock.

It is well for psychiatry to take pride in pointing to a fine record wherein a mere century has carried it out of ignorance and mysticism and out of the days when the mentally ill were whipped regularly at the full of the moon to the present era of humane treatment in modern hospitals where every facility for diagnosis and amelioration of disease is provided. In developing the curative side of psychiatry, an all-important step in advance has been the introduction of trained women nurses into all the mental wards and the placing of trained supervisors at the head of the nursing staffs. This system, first introduced by Doctor Samuel Hitch in 1841 at Gloucester Asylum in England, has been instrumental in improving the care of patients with mental disease, has engendered a better public attitude toward mental hospitals, and has done more than anything else to soften the atmosphere of tension and mystery which still lingers about the mentally disordered patient. Mental disease is thus put on a similar footing with other forms of illness and receives the same intensive study and skillful nursing as does any other problem in general medicine.

References

Beers, Clifford W.: A Mind That Found Itself, New York, 1931, Doubleday, Doran & Co.

Bromberg, Walter: The Mind of Man, New York, 1937, Harper & Brothers.

Deutsch, Albert: The Mentally Ill in America, Garden City, New York, 1933, Doubleday, Doran & Co.

Marshall, Helen E.: Dorothea Dix, Chapel Hill, 1937, University of North Carolina Press.

Ray, Marie B.: Doctors of the Mind, Boston, 1942, Little, Brown & Co.

Singer, Charles: A Short History of Medicine, New York, 1928, Oxford University Press.

Winkler, John K., and Bromberg, Walter: Mind Explorers, New York, 1939, Reynal & Hitchcock, Inc.

Zilboorg, Gregory, and Henry, George W.: A History of Medical Psychology, New York, 1941, W. W. Norton & Co.

Questions for Chapter I

Historical Review of Psychiatry

1. Did prehistoric people know anything about the brain and its function? Whence does this information come?

2. State some facts which recorded history gives us regarding the earliest hospitals for the mentally ill.

3. To what causes were mental illnesses attributed in ancient times and during the Middle Ages?

4. Discuss the inhuman methods of treatment prior to modern times.

5. Discuss some humane methods of treatment practiced in ancient times and during the Middle Ages.

6. Tell the story of the Colony of Gheel. To what do you attribute the success of the Gheel Colony?

7. In chronological manner outline the history of the care of the mentally ill in America.

8. Identify each of the following persons by stating one outstanding contribution of each to the field of psychiatry: Hippocrates, Pinel, the Tuke brothers, Benjamin Franklin, Horace Mann, Dorothea Lynde Dix, Jean Charcot, Clifford Beers, Sigmund Freud, Wagner-Jauregg, Sakel, and Samuel Hitch.

9. Locate the following: Gheel, Bethlem Hospital, Hartford Retreat, St. Elizabeth's Hospital. With what is each place associated in psychiatric history?

10. What are five outstanding treatments of mental disorders which have been introduced during the last two decades?

Chorea — a) Sydenhams — St. Vitis Dance. Onset insidious
childs' disease — jerky movements spread
into hands & other muscles + face
& voice. Sleepless, irritable — Very rarely
does death occur —
Treatment — Complete bed rest — Barbitals & Bromides

Huntington's Chorea — Hereditary — not related to
acute chorea. Also manifests
same movements — Progressive
no real treatment — End up c
mental deterioration —

Senile Chorea —
Trydiome — Medicine used for petete mal —

CHAPTER II

HEREDITY AND MENTAL DISEASE

Common sense and everyday observation of people lead one to the conclusion that some of the components of personality are inherited while others are determined by early childhood training, by disease, by certain emotional experiences, education, good or bad luck, nutrition, and many other factors which are only faintly recognized.

Heredity is a biological process whereby certain characteristics are transmitted from parent to offspring. This transmission is said to be effected by the genes, which are fine particles in the chromatin of the nucleus of the germ cell. Their number is so great, and they gather in so many millions of combinations, that inherited characteristics are not easily predictable. For a time it was believed that personality traits were inherited as units, but it was soon realized that the problem is not so simple. What appeared as a unit characteristic, such as blue eyes, black hair, or sour disposition, was found to be modified and varied in a great many directions. When Mendel, the Moravian monk, laid down his laws of heredity, it must be remembered that he began his experiments with pure strains of peas. His mathematical rules cannot entirely be applied to human beings because the latter are hopeless mixtures or hybrids. Nevertheless, Mendelian inheritance is held to be a general fact in both the plant and the animal world. Mendel found that certain characteristics are apparently represented by fairly fixed aggregations of genes and are persistently reproduced through succeeding generations; these are called *dominant* characters. An example of what may be considered a dominant characteristic is a disease known as Huntington's chorea. A family record of this disease is presented in a geneological chart, Fig. 1. Other properties fail to reappear as frequently in the offspring; they are readily "bred out" of the lineage and are known as *recessive* characters. If an individual with a recessive trait mates with a normal person, all the offspring will be normal, but, if two individuals pos-

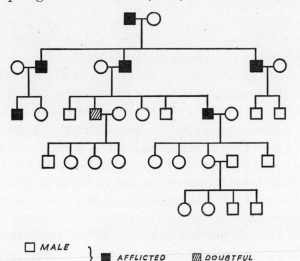

☐ MALE
◯ FEMALE } ■ AFFLICTED ▨ DOUBTFUL

Fig. 1.—Family chart of Huntington's chorea, illustrating a dominant trait. The members of the younger or later generations are not afflicted because the disease manifests itself only after midlife.

sessing the same recessive character marry and produce children, all of them will have the same recessive trait, for recessive traits breed true. For example, if a deaf-mute mates with a normal person, none of the offspring will be abnormal. If two deaf-mutes marry, they will have all deaf-mute children. Characters which may be bred out for several generations may appear again when a particular combination of genes is effected. Through such a process is explained the cropping out of an abnormal condition in a child of normal parents.

Inheritance of Intellectual and Temperamental Traits

Unlike inherited physical features, which can easily be observed, those traits called intelligence and temperament are such complex and variable phenomena that it is next to impossible to determine just what basic components are inborn or genetic and what are largely added by environmental influences. Yet only a freak combination of the genes can explain the peculiar ability of certain imbeciles to perform amazing tricks in mathematics without pencil and paper or to name the corresponding day of the week if given any day of the month within a period of twenty years. That there are inherited factors in intellect is further indicated by the fact that different races of mankind under the same environment show a clear difference in mental accomplishment. Differences in mental capacity exist in different families of the same race. Children with a high intelligence quotient generally belong to families with unusual intelligence. Exceptional artistic ability or musical endowment has been traced for three or more generations in a large number of families. Where men, like Lincoln, appear to spring from a mediocre stock, there is every reason to suppose that either too little is known of the pedigree or that extraordinary traits were latent and were the result of a happy recombination of genes.

On the temperamental side, the evidence showing hereditary factors is even more insecure. Temperament is not easy to define and even more difficult to measure in a quantitative way. In general, it is expressed by the degree of animation that is consistently demonstrated throughout life and by the social reactions of the individual. It appears that excessive activity is a dominant trait, and, when one of the parents is overactive and possesses a vigorous capacity to indulge in many social affairs, at least half the children will show the same tendency. On the other hand, when both parents are phlegmatic, the children tend to show the same torpid and sluggish disposition.

Inheritance of Mental Disease

It can be readily understood that a hyperactive trait may be exaggerated to the point that the individual reacts to situations about him with physical and vocal excess, that he may become boisterous, obtrusive, and may show marked emotional excitement. This may mean a predisposition to a so-called affective psychosis of the manic type. Likewise an individual inclined to apathy and phlegmatic disposition may deepen this tendency to a state of true depression which is also regarded as an affective disorder. We may have families characterized by such deep depression that suicides frequently occur in them. If only one of the parents has an affective psychosis, over 30 per cent of the children will have the same disorder, and in addition many more will show minor trends toward chronic excitement or mild dejection.

Another and even more common disease which displays a hereditary factor is schizophrenia, in which there seems to be a fundamental lack of certain instinctual and emotional components. If only one of the parents has this disease, over 10 per cent of the children are likewise affected and about 30 per cent may have schizophrenic tendencies. If both parents have this affliction, nearly two-thirds of the offspring are almost certain to suffer the same fate. The figures are decidedly pessimistic and become more so if one includes the data concerning the more common borderline conditions such as the psychoneuroses, where a careful study revealed that

80 per cent of the families of the persons affected showed evidence of some form of nervous disorder.

A final argument for the hereditary factor in mental disorders is found in the statistical study of the total population. It appears that such personality disorders as the affective psychoses and schizophrenia are a biologic constancy in the population, for the expectancy of affective psychoses is about 4 per cent while that of schizophrenia is 8.5 per cent.

These figures, which would argue for heredity as being such a powerful determinant in personality, may be faulty for the reason that the concept of heredity and environment is constantly being modified. If genes represent the inherited elements in personality, it should be pointed out that the individual is actually the result of these genes reacting to the surrounding cellular tissue and to the hormones or secretions in the tissue fluids, and these in turn are affected by the nutritive elements obtained from the environment. It is still a question as to what extent the health of the mother determines the personality of the offspring. Infantile diseases and the emotional relationships of the child to other members of the family are powerful determinants of personality. Sudden and radical changes in environment may drastically modify the basic elements in personality, as demonstrated by the greater frequency of mental disorder in immigrants than in the native-born of this country. All these arguments pro and con are presented to show that heredity and environment cannot be treated as unrelated factors in a sensible understanding of the innate forces in personality and its disorders.

There are only a few permissible conclusions on heredity in mental disease, and these can be stated as follows:

Psychopathic parents seem to have more abnormal children than do normal parents.

Certain families are notable for having a high frequency of mental disorders. Manic-depressive psychoses have a particular disposition to familial incidence.

In general, manic-depressive insanity appears to be a dominant trait while schizophrenia appears to follow a recessive course.

While feeblemindedness and epilepsy are said to be inherited, when such conditions appear in a single offspring, this does not necessarily indicate that there is a familial degeneracy. A really bad stock is one which consistently manifests a wide range of stigmata such as was demonstrated in the notorious Kallikak family, and which expressed themselves as criminality, prostitution, alcoholism, epilepsy, feeblemindedness, as well as insanity.

References

Association for Research in Nervous and Mental Diseases: Heredity in Nervous and Mental Disease, New York, 1923, Paul B. Hoeber, Inc.

Eugenical Sterilization: Report of the Committee of the American Neurological Association for the Investigation of Eugenical Sterilization, New York, 1936, The Macmillan Company.

Jennings, H. S.: The Biological Basis of Human Nature, New York, 1930, W. W. Norton & Co.

Questions for Chapter II
Heredity and Mental Disease

1. Name several factors which may affect the personality.
2. What is heredity and by what mechanism does it operate?
3. Who was Mendel? What basic observation did he make?
4. Are inherited traits usually predictable? Explain.
5. What is meant by a "dominant character"? Give an example.
6. What is meant by a "recessive character"? Give an example.
7. What facts indicate that there are inherited factors in intellect?
8. What, in general, is meant by temperament?
9. Name two mental diseases which display hereditary trends.
10. In what manner do population statistics support the hereditary concept of mental disease?

CHAPTER III

THE STRUCTURE OF PERSONALITY

The term personality is loosely and freely used, and to different people it often connotes different ideas. In general, it means the aggregate of the physical and mental qualities in any person as these respond in characteristic fashion to different situations. Such distinguish the individual from others and give him his own peculiar identity. It is the person as he is known to his friends.

The ingredients which make up adult personality are many; some are hard to define and are often merely sensed in a vague way. Personality development is a complex and dynamic process which must be studied by many different methods of approach. No two human beings are exactly alike at birth, and no two human beings have had an exactly identical experience with life.

The Instinctual Components in Personality

The fundamental need of all animal life is action. This action is the outward expression of inborn forces which are commonly called instincts. This reservoir of energy which compels certain modes of action is common to both man and animal and is called the *libido*.

There are probably only two basic channels through which this energy can be expressed, one which assures or attempts to secure preservation of life by getting food and the other to promote perpetuation of the species, in short, the instincts of *hunger* and *sex*. Perhaps a third primordial one is the *herd* instinct. In a pure state, that is without modification, instincts are really unconscious or reflex-like reactions without any clear recognition of the end to be obtained; yet they are indispensable because they have a life and death value in the evolution of the race.

While instincts in themselves are not conscious in their operation, certain experiences associated with them called feelings or *emotions* are definitely conscious. Thus, if the satisfaction or free expression of an instinct is allowed, this is accompanied by a feeling of pleasure, and, if the instinct is frustrated or inhibited, the feeling is one of displeasure or general discomfort.

At birth in man the instincts have but a few simple means of expression; but these multiply and become elaborated into complex patterns, for environment and growth greatly modify them, particularly in the human being. Hunger is quickly expressed in the newborn infant in the sucking reflex, and it is easily satisfied. The sex instinct, however, has a slow development and one peculiarly its own, for according to Freud it passes through several stages before it completely ripens in the adult. It is present at birth, but the object or person upon which it consciously desires to focus changes from stage to stage. First of all, the instinct gains satisfaction in early infancy by giving the child a pleasurable feeling when various parts of its body are manipulated by the mother. The infant may also derive this pleasure by active participation in such acts as nursing, thumbsucking, and defecation, thereby stimulating his own erotic zones. Somewhere in the same level of development the sex instinct may select the person himself as a love object, and we have the *narcissistic* or "I-love-me" stage. In the next stage the object becomes another person but of the same sex, and here the growing child finds free expression of this instinct in play and social activities with one of his own kind—hence the *homosexual* stage. Finally, the matured instinct focuses

Super-ego — Unconscious conscience acts as inhibitor — [handwritten annotation at top of page]

its full force upon individuals of the opposite sex, and the final or *heterosexual* stage is achieved. This last stage not only implies adult sex instinct, but also involves the parental instinct which inspires home building and promotes the formation of the family group.

Freud has further propounded that this development of sex instinct may be arrested at any stage, and such immaturity is regarded as one of the prime causes of inadequate personality, poor adaptation to life's problems, and failure in family and marriage relations.

Probably allied to the hunger and self-preservation instincts are those reactions which bring forth the emotions of fear and rage. There is an innate tendency in every human being to respond to dangerous situations either by running away or fighting. A position of security prompts an aggressive, pugnacious response, while, on the other hand, if the hazards are too great, flight is the usual reaction. Both fear and anger are complicated, but fairly uniform, physiological phenomena in man, involving a large portion of the nervous system and setting up responses in glands, blood vessels, and other viscera in the body. A feeling of inferiority is in a sense a chronic fear and may be a vital factor in deciding whether or not personality shall be efficient and successful.

Obviously every instinct cannot find free satisfaction at all times. Satisfaction must be frequently delayed or achieved in a devious way until certain conditions in the environment have been fulfilled. This ability to postpone satisfaction is the function of *consciousness*. When the instinct rises into the conscious mind, it appears as a wish which is directed on an object. As long as the wish remains unsatisfied, there is a tension. This is discharged in a motor act which attempts to obtain the object.

[handwritten notes in top margin: Id activates or motivates our actions thru unconsciousness! Ego - acts as arbitrator between Id & Super Ego — Intelligence —]

Some instinctual wants are not easily satisfied because society regards them as distasteful. The individual is, therefore, ashamed of possessing such wants. In other words, the person finds himself harboring two different instinctual forces pulling in different directions. One instinct prompts him to seek satisfaction through an act; another equally strong prompts him to maintain the esteem of others. Therefore there are a conflict and a tension which cannot be easily discharged. This tension becomes a form of nervousness and illness. The person may then try to "forget" or disown his distasteful cravings. What actually happens is that he does not forget them, he forcibly represses them into the unconscious. The ideas thus denounced are all held together by a strong emotional bond and are known as a *complex*. Complexes are not all abnormal. Sometimes they obtain expression in various constructive and helpful activities, a process which is called sublimation. A complex becomes harmful when it remains repressed in the unconscious for a long time. There this repressed energy or wish is no longer under the direct control of consciousness or of the will and may find expression in fantastic wish-fulfillment, in excessive preoccupation with self, and in queer physical symptoms.

This tendency to direct the instinctual energy into one's inner mental life is called *introversion*. The more natural trend is to direct psychic energy upon the world of reality and to be more quickly reactive to one's environment, a quality of personality called *extroversion*.

The structure of personality according to the Freudian concept consists of three main divisions:

a. **The Id.**—The instinctual and unconscious levels where are repressed the primary drives and from whence comes all psychic energy.

b. **The Ego.**—The conscious levels of personality which are represented by the strictly intellectual and volitional features. It is that portion of the personality which the individual presents to the outside world, the "showcase" of personality.

c. **The Superego.**—The voice of conscience or that phase of personality which is keenly sensitive to the demands of strict convention and which acts as a strong inhibitor of the id.

Personality and Body Build

Since ancient times attempts have been made to classify human beings according to physique and mental characteristics. For instance, the Hindus distinguished three types of man, called symbolically the hare, the bull, and the horse. In folk-philosophy the virtuous people were usually portrayed as long lean individuals with pointed noses, narrow chins, and sad countenances. Fat people with stolid bodies are generally presented as jolly, harmless, and comic creatures. Kretschmer, a German psychiatrist, correlated physique and mental characteristics after careful psychological and physical measurements. He divides people into three main body types, which he calls the asthenic, athletic, and pyknic.

The asthenic person is tall, lean, and flat chested and has a long oval head. His temperament, likely to be shy, introverted, emotionally cold, methodical and sensitive, is called **schizothymic**.

The **pyknic** type is short, stocky, compact, round chested, square or round headed, and the disposition which commonly goes with this body build is extroverted, sociable, aggressive, and expansive, but is inclined to wide swings in mood. Hence he is termed syntonic or **cyclothymic**, and, if mental breakdown occurs, it is likely to be a manic-depressive psychosis.

The **athletic** type is in a manner of speaking halfway between the asthenic and pyknic. He has a large muscular build, broad shoulders, and graceful tapering limbs. His temperament lies between the schizothymic and cyclothymic.

None of these typings of human beings are absolute. There are so many combinations and variations in both physique and temperament that any constitutional classification should be accepted as a very general one. Probably the above types are simply the extreme deviations in personality forms.

The Brain and Personality

Attempts have been frequently made to interpret personality in terms of function of various parts of the central nervous system. About a century ago before there was much knowledge of brain function, some rather ludicrous ideas were advanced by which various attributes of personality were assigned to certain prominences or "bumps" on the skull and to certain folds of the brain cortex. This pseudoscience is called phrenology.

The brain and cord are the master organs for coordinating all bodily activities, but the relation of their functions to specific personality traits is not well understood. Except in some organic brain diseases, there is no clear knowledge of what changes occur in the nerve tissues in most personality disorders.

The functions of each major portion of the brain have been investigated, but their individual contributions to the total personality are known only in a general way. The most effective method of presenting the organic background of personality is to describe each division of the central nervous system beginning with the less complicated and more primitive parts.

The Spinal Cord.—This is essentially a conducting cable containing nerve tracks passing up to the brain and passing from the higher centers to the various nerve trunks of the body. In its gray matter the cord contains nerve cells which provide for the simplest defensive movements. These are automatic, fixed motor patterns which are also present in the lowest form of mammal life.

The Medulla.—This is really nothing more than an upward extension of the spinal cord. It is responsible for the special reflex activities of the throat, such as coughing, sneezing, swallowing, and gagging. Its greatest importance lies in the fact that it vitally controls respiration and heart action.

The Pons and Cerebellum are structures which concern themselves largely with muscular coordination in securing balance and tone to offset the forces of gravity. They do not contribute a very prominent component to personality except in a purely physical sense.

The Midbrain.—Here reside the centers for coordinating the special sensations of sight and hearing and those which account for pupillary, ocular, and auditory reflex movements. Although this part of the brain is very small, it contains the red nuclei which have much to do in controlling the common automatic movements necessary in walking, turning, and running.

The Diencephalon.—This portion of the brain is relatively simple in structure; yet in some complicated manner it probably is the main source of all the instinctual mechanisms which give personality its basic properties.

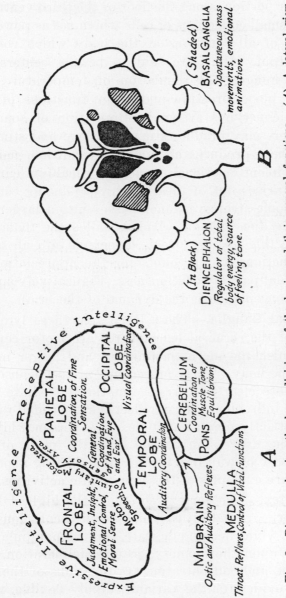

Fig. 2.—Diagram showing the large divisions of the brain and their general functions. (*A*) A lateral view demonstrating the main lobes of the cerebrum and the important structures in the brain stem. (*B*) A cross section presenting the deep-seated structures such as the diencephalon and the motor basal ganglia.

In its lower portion, along the floor of the third ventricle, are found small collections of cells which act as powerful regulators of all functions of the body which control energy output. Here are said to be the centers for sleep, for hunger, for regulation of temperature, for control of blood pressure and other functions of the sympathetic nervous system. Stimulation of some of these centers may produce stupor or sleep and stimulation of others produces an opposite condition, namely rage and violent emotional tension. Probably a current of feeling arises out of these energy-producing centers which in some strange manner passes into a larger nucleus in the diencephalon which is called the thalamus. From here this feeling tone is dispersed into all other mental functions and accounts for the appreciation of the emotional part of consciousness. Figuratively speaking, the diencephalon is the dynamo of the brain.

The Basal Ganglia.—These large structures lying at the base of the cerebral hemispheres are motor centers which furnish the more spontaneous and larger movements of the body. These movements are semiconscious and are more clearly expressive of the immediate feelings of the individual. They reflect the emotional rather than the strictly mental attitudes of a person while in action. The expression on the face, the poise of the body, the ease of walking, turning and shifting about of the limbs are examples of these automatic activities.

The Cortex.—The cortex represents the highest level of behavior. All activities which require conscious coordination, which demand delicate, skillful manipulation, which call upon the memory, require deliberation, discrimination, and concentration are functions of the cortex. It provides for the variable, highly flexible, more elaborate responses to stimuli from the environment.

Examples of these delicate, highly developed functions are speech and the remarkably adept movements of the hands.

The cortex is anatomically subdivided into several large areas or lobes which, however, never act independently but associate their functions with those of all other parts of the brain.

The parietal lobe or area is chiefly concerned with receiving the finer discriminative sensations, particularly from the hand, which are elaborated to allow concepts of shape, form and accurate location of stimuli or objects. Defects in this area result in a numb, clumsy, or useless hand.

The occipital area receives optic sensations and brings into consciousness visual images. In man this area is particularly developed to utilize the word as a symbol of the image so that reading as a cortical function is possible.

The temporal lobe is concerned mainly with the function of hearing. Auditory impressions become invested with meaning so that the spoken word is understood.

Around the sylvian fissure the special sensory impressions brought in from the hand, the eye, and the ear are further associated and elaborated and the combination of all these functions becomes receptive intelligence. Impressions are amplified and stored as memory phenomena.

About the rolandic fissure are found the motor centers which convey to the muscles of the body those combinations of stimuli which result in the many fine manipulations of the hand for skillful acts and of the tongue and lips for speech. Here reside the motor centers for all highly volitional activity.

The frontal lobe is the center for all the final correlations of the brain and assumes therefore a superior position. The ultimate integration of personality probably depends upon the frontal lobe. It determines to what degree reason shall dominate emotion; how well the individual is able to draw upon his intellectual experiences to dictate his judgment, his insight, and his moral behavior. It makes possible the highest degree of reasoning in terms of the abstract and away from the instinctual and emotional trends. In short it represents the noblest and highest attributes of personality. Because of its heavy responsibilities and its delicate structure, it is more prone to injury and disease. Any serious defect in its function is at once manifested by personality changes, by a blunting of moral sense, and by a tendency to behavior which is dominated by emotion rather than by judgment and reason.

· References

Berry, R. J. A.: Your Brain and Its Story, New York, 1939, Oxford University Press.

Campbell, Charles M.: Human Personality and Environment, New York, 1934, The Macmillan Co.

Cobb, Stanley: A Preface to Nervous Disease, Baltimore, 1936, William Wood & Co.

Cobb, Stanley: Borderlands of Psychiatry, Cambridge, Mass., 1943, Harvard University Press.

Douglas, A. C.: The Physical Mechanism of the Human Mind, Edinburgh, 1932, E. & S. Livingstone.

Freud, Sigmund: New Introductory Lectures on Psychoanalysis, translated by W. J. H. Sprott, New York, 1933, W. W. Norton & Co., Inc.

Herrick, C. Judson: The Thinking Machine, Chicago, 1929, The University of Chicago Press.

Kretschmer, E.: Physique and Character, translated by W. J. H. Sprott, New York, 1925, Harcourt, Brace & Co., Inc.

Wertheimer and Hesketh: The Significance of the Physical Constitution in Mental Disease, Medicine Monographs Vol. X, Baltimore, 1926, Williams & Wilkins Co.

Wolff, Werner: The Expression of Personality, New York, 1943, Harper & Brothers.

Questions for Chapter III
The Structure of Personality

1. Define personality in a general way.
2. What are the three basic instincts of the human race? Are these instincts conscious reactions? Why couldn't we get along without them?
3. Discuss the Freudian theory of the development of the sex instinct from the time of birth until maturity is reached.
4. Give an explanation of what might happen if this development is arrested at any one of the stages named.
5. What may cause the experienced emotions of fear and rage? Describe both the psychological and the physical aspects of these emotions.
6. What is the function of consciousness?
7. Define the following terms: id, ego, and superego.
8. Give the psychological and physical characteristics of each of the following types of personality: the asthenic, the pyknic, the athletic. Can most persons be classified as being strictly one type or another? What psychiatrist made this classification?
9. Which of the following terms are related to each other: asthenic, syntonic, schizothymic, cyclothymic and pyknic.
10. Name the various parts of the central nervous system and state the function or functions of each part. Why is it important to know the function of each part of the central nervous system when studying personality?

CHAPTER IV

DEFENSE MECHANISMS OF PERSONALITY

Since the deep instinctual forces of the human being are the sources of psychic energy and since some of these forces are frequently in conflict with each other thus giving rise to tension and nervousness, the human being resorts to certain devices by means of which this tension may be relieved. These mental tricks are employed by all people to a certain degree, but under abnormal stress they may become very prominent characteristics and may stamp the individual as neurotic or grossly abnormal.

In a sense these devices or *mental dynamisms,* as they are often called, are compromises with forbidden desires, feelings of guilt, or an admission that one is inadequate in facing certain problems. They serve to salvage the ego or pride, avoid an open exposure of failure, and save psychic energy. Only a few of the more commonly utilized dynamisms will be presented.

Rationalization.—This is a mental device which is almost universally employed. It is useful when one has a sense of guilt about something one does or believes, or when one is a little uncertain about his behavior. It is simply a device whereby one attempts to make his behavior appear to be the result of logical thinking, rather than the result of unconscious desires or cravings. In court we unconsciously testify in favor of our friends. We try to make our religious convictions logical; we argue with self-righteousness that our political beliefs are based on fact. We cover up our mistakes and failures by explaining them away in terms of unavoidable misfortune and hopefully trust that others will ac-

46

cept such explanations. In short, any explanation which is recognized as an "alibi" is regarded as a rationalization.

Sublimation.—By this device primitive cravings and impulses which are ordinarily repressed gain outward expression by converting their energies into socially accepted activities. A woman who has been deprived of an opportunity to express her sexual and maternal instincts through marriage may gratify them by becoming a teacher. A young lover may convert his burning but unrequited love into music or poetry. The young woman with a great urge to display her physical charms may sublimate this exhibitionistic instinct in dancing on the public stage. Scientific curiosity is said to be a sublimation of the early sexual curiosity formerly satisfied by peeping through keyholes. Sublimation is, therefore, believed to be responsible for the major portion of the great artistic and cultural achievements of all civilized peoples.

Repression.—Memories of disagreeable impressions, shameful experiences or impulses are forcibly dismissed from consciousness, and the psychic energy with which they were loaded becomes part of the unconscious. The more acute the conscience the more material will be thus repressed, particularly matters which deal with the sex impulse. Hence, the selfish and hostile impulses become most frequently repressed, and such repression always means internal conflict. The repressed material may find escape through conversion into physical defects, into obsessions, and into morbid anxiety which arises without apparent reason.

Projection.—By this dynamism a person overcomes his feeling of inadequacy and guilt by transferring to others the responsibility for such inadequacy. The guilty one feels less guilty by assigning his misdemeanors to others. The unfaithful husband placates his conscience by believing his wife is untrue. The paranoiac, shameful of his own inner hate of others, feels relieved by entertaining ideas that others are plotting against him. The voice of his own conscience is projected as if coming from others, and he, therefore, hears voices (hallucinations) talking in disparaging terms about him. The paranoid individual, therefore, desires to believe in his persecutions and cannot be cured by convincing him of his errors in belief.

Identification.—In a manner of speaking this mechanism is the exact opposite to projection. By this device we attach and transfer to our own ego certain qualities or desirable elements found in the personality of another or in objects in the outside world. A psychotic patient who believes he is Christ lets his beard and hair grow long. A young interne who admires his senior surgeon who has a habit of wearing a rose in his lapel will adorn himself with the same flower. A butler who serves a distinguished personage feels greatly superior to other servants whose masters are not so distinguished. Another form of identification is that wherein one may have an unreasoning sympathy for an offender because of a common unconscious sense of guilt.

Compensation.—Here feelings of guilt or inferiority are so strong that they prompt defensive reactions that are excessive. A man who is tormented by his physical weaknesses reacts by becoming overaggressive, by indulging in violent exercise, and by pursuing a career wherein he is allowed to display his virility. A youth who is tormented by the shame of living in a drunkard's household becomes a prominent prohibitionist in later life. In an exhilarated state a person may make wild and grandiose pronouncements and claims which reveal his failures and inadequacies of the present. Most compensations are believed to be largely motivated by a sense of sexual inadequacy. Men who are sexual weaklings may compensate by resentment and abuse of their womenfolk.

Conversion.—Disagreeable experiences and shameful desires when repressed into the unconscious may reappear as physical symptoms, but the patient is unaware of any connection between the two phenomena. Thus, a child who is torn by a conflict arising out of a chronic friction between her parents whom she loves may find herself suddenly blind so that she may not look upon such incompatibility. A young girl who fears that she must make an accounting of her misbehavior to her parents suddenly develops a paralysis of her vocal cords. The conversion is not always so simple and frequently it is difficult to determine just what conflicts in the repressed unconscious produce a certain physical defect, but always the disability serves to distract attention from the real problems. Conversion is a dynamism particularly useful to the person who is prone to hysteria.

Symbolization and Condensation.—Instinctual desires may announce themselves through symbols, the meaning of which is not exactly clear to the conscious mind, for these symbols are the language of the unconscious. Such symbols appear in dreams, in fantasies and may emerge through various rituals or obsessive behavior.

Symbols may become further merged by condensation to represent a wide range of emotionally painful ideas which thus become lumped together so as to lose their painful significance. When they arise to the conscious levels, they are emitted as an apparently incoherent jumble of words whose real meanings are hidden in the unconscious. Such condensations of thinking are frequently noted in the language of the schizophrenic patient, which may be irrational to the doctor and the nurse, but to the patient, himself, are full of meaning and coherency.

Displacement.—Frequently it is impossible to give free expression to some impulses or feelings, and this frustration is relieved by discharging the feelings upon some entirely different situation. The man who is cringing under the insults and denunciations of his employer may come home and kick his dog to relieve his feelings. Painful preoccupation with the sexual organs may be displaced to other viscera whose disorders can be discussed with propriety. An individual with some deep conflict between instincts may displace this warfare from his own emotional spheres and transfer it to a boxing contest in which he feels himself as one contender who must vanquish the other. A very common instance of displacement is the sudden impulse to get to a certain place before a certain time, as the thought, "If I don't get to the street corner by the stroke of eight o'clock something terrible may happen to me." In this situation the person transfers his tension from some insoluble and perplexing problem to the race against time, which, if won, at least momentarily relieves his tension.

All these peculiar strategies are found in nervous and mental patients, and represent an attempt on the part of the personality in distress to maintain self-esteem and self-security. They are of great significance to the psychopathologist and should be of interest to the nurse who is desirous of observing how personality maintains its integrity against total collapse. These alibis or compromises when displayed to a marked degree indicate serious maladjustment and frequently appear as a warning of more disastrous events to come. To detect their presence in early personality disorder and to correct the situations which prompt them is probably one of the most essential measures in preventing total disorganization of the personality.

References

Freud, Sigmund: The Basic Writings of Sigmund Freud, translated and edited by A. A. Brill, New York, 1938, The Modern Library.

Henry, George W.: Essentials of Psychopathology, Baltimore, William Wood & Co.

Malamud, William: Outlines of General Psychopathology, New York, 1935, W. W. Norton & Co., Inc.

Strecker, Edward A.: Beyond the Clinical Frontiers, New York, 1940, W. W. Norton & Co., Inc.

White, William Allen: Essays in Psychopathology, Nervous and Mental Disease Monographs, New York.

Questions on Chapter IV

Defense Mechanisms of Personality

1. Describe the dynamism of "rationalization."
2. Describe the mechanism of "sublimation." Is it a desirable mechanism?
3. Explain the mechanism of "repression." The impulses most frequently repressed are of what nature? In what form may these repressed impulses escape?
4. Explain the mechanism of "projection." In what mental illness is this demonstrated?
5. Describe the "identification" mechanism. Give some examples to illustrate its meaning.
6. Make clear the meaning of "compensation." What instinct is believed to motivate most compensations?
7. Describe the "conversion" mechanism, and give some examples to illustrate its meaning.
8. Explain the mechanisms of "symbolization" and "condensation." Give examples of each.
9. Describe the mechanism of "displacement."
10. Why should the nurse understand these dynamisms and their significance?

CHAPTER V

THE CAUSES AND CLASSIFICATION OF MENTAL DISEASES

While other branches of medicine deal with specific organs of the body, psychiatry studies the individual as a whole, as he is engaged with varying degrees of success in adjusting himself to his environment and as this environment, in turn, affects him. No one set of facts are taken into consideration when looking for the causes of mental breakdown, but the integrated facts of all biology—anatomical, physiologic, pathologic, and psychological—must be studied before we are to understand human behavior, both normal and abnormal. This broad approach to the etiology and understanding of mental disorders is called the *psychobiological* concept and constitutes the most modern and most promising one, because it implies a constructive and hopeful attitude toward therapy and readjustment of the mentally ill patient.

Very much like the psychobiology of Dr. Meyer which studies the "whole human being in difficulty" is the new approach termed *psychosomatic medicine* which serves the purpose of reminding one of the ever-present connections between bodily and mental functioning. Abnormal personality reactions may provoke abnormal function of body organs, and disturbed organic function may cause mental disorders. The effect of strong emotions on such conditions as duodenal ulcer, hypertension, coronary heart disease, and goiter is closely studied. This interlocking of mind and body clearly shows the absurdity of the notion that psychologic illness is one thing and physical disorder another.

Even such a specific disease of the brain as syphilis, with its fairly characteristic pathology, cannot adequately explain all the behavior difficulties which accompany such changes. In varying degrees this behavior will be colored by the innate temperament of the patient, by his peculiar instinctual make-up as well as his own particular emotional and mental attitudes which have been conditioned by experiences which he had long before the brain disease developed. Every mental disorder is an individual problem which can be fully understood only after a study of the whole personality and of those hereditary, physical, mental, emotional, and instinctual elements which go to make up that personality.

Heredity.—Just how much contribution heredity makes to the causation of mental disease has already been discussed in a previous chapter. In general, it can be said that it is an important factor, but its influence has probably been overemphasized. Only a few rare forms of mental disease are known to be definitely transmitted according to the Mendelian ratio. The disposition to manic-depressive psychosis is probably an inherited one. General enfeeblement which consistently expresses itself in the family stock as idiocy, epilepsy, mental disease, and physical infirmity undoubtedly can be laid to a deficiency in the germ cell. Moreover, offspring of depleted stock are likely to meet a greater handicap in the poor environmental setting in which their inefficient parents put them. Because these two factors are so frequently and so hopelessly intermingled, our conclusions as to the strict hereditary causes of mental disease must remain subject to revision.

The Age Factor.—Young children rarely show a frank mental disease, but the incidence rises sharply at the beginning of adolescence. At this age level the all-important adjustment of the individual to external social influences and to internal sexual strivings is apparently responsible for intrapsychic tensions which often result in disorganization of the personality. This may be the most important contributing cause in many of the schizophrenias which develop so frequently at this critical age.

The menopause or the involutional period may likewise be an underlying factor, for it is also one of the "tides of life" when mental breakdown is frequent, not only because of the declining activity of the reproductive organs, but because of the disappointments, life failures, and other frustrations which become painfully evident at this time. People are wont to look upon midlife as a time when life's work should be well established, a milestone at which one must make an accounting. Spinsters look upon it as a turn in life when marriage no longer is possible; married women fear it because it marks a decline and opens the dread vista of impending old age.

Old age itself is unquestionably a prime factor in mental disease, for it is the age of cerebral arteriosclerosis and brain atrophy as well as a period of increasing difficulty in economic and social matters. The specter of the poorhouse is a not uncommon source of agitation and anxiety in the aged. In the last quarter century the number of old people with cerebral arteriosclerosis admitted to New York state hospitals increased sixfold. This is partly due to the fact that more people live long enough to acquire the mental infirmities of old age, and more old people find themselves financially destitute and break down because they cannot successfully meet the psychological situations which arise as a result of economic and social insecurity.

Alcohol.—Alcoholism may at once be a cause and a symptom of mental disease. Usually it is taken because it offers a "flight from reality," and the frequent use of alcohol implies an inability to face a disagreeable situation with confidence or to compensate for a deficiency, such as homosexuality. When the person is moderately intoxicated to the point of exhilaration, the desires and strivings of the individual are permitted to come to the surface and to be freely expressed. Alcohol may be taken in excess to cover a period of depression or moroseness in a cyclothymic person. In another type of personality, various intrapersonality tensions are exposed through hallucinations and delusional states. In chronic alcoholism the brain suffers injury, and there is a progressive disintegration of the personality with characteristic physical and mental changes. There is a direct relation between the amount of alcohol consumed in a given community and the number of mental cases of alcoholic origin occurring in that community.

Other Drugs.—While alcohol is the most common intoxicant taken habitually, other drugs are resorted to by unstable and maladjusted persons for the same general reason, namely, to dull the sensorium and to escape from the trying ordeals of life. All of these produce this desired effect and in larger doses bring on mental dullness, stupidity, coma, and even delirium. The most frequent agents causing these mental changes are morphine, cocaine, bromides, barbituric acid derivatives, and marihuana. In chronic drug addiction there is the same deterioration of personality one finds in the degenerated alcoholic.

Syphilis.—Syphilitic disease of the brain accounts for nearly ten per cent of all admissions to state hospitals in this country. It is far more frequent in men than in women, and is more prevalent in the larger cities. It is definitely an acquired disease, but a small number of cases are found to be of the congenital type. Whether syphilis plays an important role in hereditary transmission of constitutional deficiency without actual infection is an open question.

Focal Infection.—Several years ago the theory was advocated that hidden infections in the teeth, tonsils, sinuses, colon, and prostate produce toxins which affect the nervous system and produce mental disease. Surgical removal of these sites was believed to increase the recovery rate, but this hypothesis has not stood the test of experience and except in a few localities is now rejected.

Encephalitis.—Inflammation of the brain, particularly by the so-called viruses, such as occurred in the wake of the influenza epidemic in 1918, causes specific pathology and leads to various psychic and physical disorders. In its acute form it is characterized by lethargy (hence the term "sleeping sickness"), by delirium, confusion, and stupor. In its chronic form it is recognized by the clinical picture of shaking palsy or parkinsonism associated with increasing irritability, insomnia, and neurotic behavior.

Endocrine Glands.—No definite relationship has been found between malfunction of the ductless glands and mental disease except in growing children in whom the endocrine organs are congenitally absent or deficient. Most popular is the idea that excessive thyroid activity leads to a psychosis. In the vast majority of cases, where mental disease is found associated with hyperthyroidism, the trouble lies in some innate temperamental or emotional level and is often a typical mental upset such as one finds in patients who have no thyroid disturbance. Even in hypothyroidism or myxedema, where there is always a mental sluggishness or depression, many of the symptoms are those determined by the peculiar structure of the personality.

Fatigue and Overwork.—These two factors were formerly considered to be the most important causes of mental illness. One heard much of the "strain and stress of life" and "the modern tempo of living." It appears to be an "honorable" justification for mental breakdown, but actually in most instances covers up the true causes, which are mental conflicts and emotional problems. For overwork is commonly a symptom, not a cause. The individual goes into a frenzy of overwork to forget his troubles and to "keep his mind occupied," an expression which implies that the mind is incapable of solving a deep-seated personal problem. There is no fatigue like the fatigue of one whose life is insecure, whose instincts are thwarted, and whose incentive is lacking. There is no justification for the belief that the pace of modern life is responsible for a great increase in the number of mental breakdowns.

Trauma.—Injury to the head must be accepted as a potent cause of mental disturbance. If trauma is severe, particularly in cases of concussion and unconsciousness, the aftereffects may become serious and insidious degeneration may follow, often associated with epilepsy. Much more frequently, however, the physician encounters a "nervousness" which the patient assigns to an injury whether it be to the head or elsewhere. It is always difficult to determine how much of this can be attributed to true nerve injury.

Constitutional Factors.—When we speak of constitutional factors in mental disease, we have in mind a vague concept of human types wherein certain predispositions or potentialities are dictated by the physical and temperamental trends of the patient. Kretschmer has particu larly pointed out that people with a short, stocky or *pyknic* physique, characterized by a barrel-shaped torso and one given to obesity, have a lively and sociable nature, are subject to fluctuations of mood, and are at all times predictable and appropriate in their responses to external situations. From this psychophysical structure are recruited the manic-depressive psychoses. On the other hand, individuals with the so-called *asthenic* type of body, that is, with long, narrow flat trunk, thin neck, and lean, bony limbs are prone to be temperamentally shy, sensitive, aloof, cold, and somewhat jerky in their instinctual expressions. Such people adjust poorly, withdraw into abstractions and into their own inner ruminations, and under stress may develop schizophrenia.

These classifications merely indicate certain tendencies and do not apply to all individuals, for there are an endless number of variations and composites. It must be conceded, however, that there exists some fundamental correlation between body build and certain psychological types. Manic-depressive psychosis is found to be preponderantly in the person of pyknic physique, and the average schizophrenic patient is likely to be more on the thin, asthenic side in physical make-up.

These basic temperamental tendencies toward two opposite poles of variation are further expounded by Jung in his classification of human beings into the *extrovert* and *introvert*. This division into two types is determined by the general direction into which psychic energy is guided by the individual. The extrovert directs his interests to the outside world and is in keen contact with persons and affairs about him—in every sense a realist. The introvert lives within his own little shell, tends to be subjective in his interests, and shrinks from the problems of a workaday world.

Mental Factors.—Much as the physician and the nurse would have it otherwise, in the light of our present knowledge of mental disease, purely mental factors probably remain as the most common exciting causes of mental disorder. Hence, the vast majority of these disturbances are *psychogenic*. Such causes are many, but they can all be reduced to situations which give rise to a sense of insecurity, to an injury to self-esteem, to a feeling of guilt, or to an overwhelming sense of inferiority. Financial worries, troubles in domestic affairs, deep disappointments in personal relations and the sudden death of a relative are frequently revealed as critical causes. Conflict between instinctual forces within the individual himself known as *intrapsychic conflict* may break to the surface as an acute psychosis.

As indicated in a previous chapter, a conflict may exist over a long period of time between those desires dictated by the ideals and social conscience, on the one hand, and the unconscious impulses and strivings arising out of the instinctual levels, on the other. The psychosis may be just an expression of a final and ultimate method of satisfying the warring elements in personality.

The Classification of Mental Disease

No classification of mental disease is entirely satisfactory, for it has been pointed out that a mental disorder can be but rarely attributed to one specific cause. Moreover, the actual causes of many of these disturbances are but vaguely recognized. The classification which has met with the most widespread approval is that of Kraepelin, and this is largely based on the symptoms manifested by each disease. Somewhat modified to meet the practical requirements of today, this classification is used by American psychiatrists. For practical purposes and for a quick review of the subject as required by the average curriculum in nurses' training schools, it is best to follow a simpler general scheme. The one offered by Meyer which regards mental disorders as different types of reaction is probably most applicable and will be followed.

1. Affective-Reaction Types
    a. Manic-depressive psychoses
    b. Involutional psychoses
2. Schizophrenic Reaction Types
3. Paranoid Reaction Types
4. Reaction Types With Somatic Disease
    a. Symptomatic psychoses
    b. Psychoses with endocrine disease
5. Delirious Reaction Types
    a. Alcoholic psychoses
    b. Drug psychoses
6. Organic Reaction Types
    a. Psychoses with syphilis of the central nervous system
    b. Traumatic psychoses
    c. Psychoses with brain tumor and other brain disease
    d. Psychoses with cerebral arteriosclerosis
    e. Senile psychoses
7. Epilepsy and Psychoses With Epilepsy
8. Mental Deficiency
9. Psychopathic Personality
10. The Psychoneuroses
    a. Neurasthenia
    b. Anxiety state
    c. Hysteria
    d. Psychasthenia
11. Other Psychoses

References

Billings, Edward G.: A Handbook of Elementary Psychobiology and Psychiatry, New York, 1939, The Macmillan Co.

Henderson and Gillespie: A Textbook of Psychiatry, New York, 1927, Oxford University Press.

Muncie, Wendell: Psychobiology and Psychiatry, St. Louis, 1939, The C. V. Mosby Company.

Richards, Esther L.: Introduction to Psychobiology and Psychiatry, St. Louis, 1941, The C. V. Mosby Co.

Weiss, Edward, and English, O. Spurgeon: Psychosomatic Medicine, Phila., 1943, W. B. Saunders Co.

Questions for Chapter V

The Causes and Classification of Mental Diseases

1. What is meant by the psychobiological concept of the study of human behavior?
2. What relationship is emphasized by psychosomatic medicine in the study of human illness? Give examples.
3. Why is it difficult to draw conclusions as to strict hereditary causes of most mental diseases?
4. Name three age factors which may be instrumental in causing mental disease. Discuss each factor.
5. Name the habit-forming intoxicants or drugs most frequently taken. Which is the most common one?
6. What type of people resort to drugs and alcohol? For what purpose? May alcoholism be a symptom rather than a disease?
7. What part does syphilis play in the causation of mental disease? It is most prevalent in which sex and in what localities? Can this disease be congenital?
8. Discuss the relationship between mental diseases and each of the following: focal infections, encephalitis, endocrine glands, fatigue, overwork, and trauma.
9. What is meant by the term "psychogenic"?
10. What are the most common exciting causes of mental disorders?
11. Whose classification of mental diseases are we using in this text? Are there other classifications?

CHAPTER VI

THE EXAMINATION OF THE MENTAL PATIENT

The understanding of human behavior is a complicated subject, for it must include an inquiry into every remote phase of the individual's life history, some of it involving very intimate and personal matters. This longitudinal study of the patient's personality through space and time, together with a knowledge of the immediate mental and physical state, constitutes the psychobiological method of recognizing the nature of mental disorder.

The complete examination of a mental patient can be conveniently divided into three major parts: (1) the examination of the patient's life history, (2) the direct examination of the patient as he presents himself at the time of illness, and (3) the data obtained from observation of the patient at home or in an institution.

The Life History of the Patient

The vast majority of mental disorders are a final resultant or culmination of numerous factors which have existed for various periods of time in the personality of the patient. What these factors may be can best be demonstrated by a systematic inquiry into the patient's complete life record up to the time of the present illness. This information should be gleaned from as many sources as possible and particularly from those whose point of view is not too biased or distorted.

The following components are most valuable in compiling significant data:

1. Family History:
   Feeblemindedness, epilepsy, alcohol, insanity, syphilis. Parents', sisters' and brothers' temperament and physical condition. *usual childhood diseases*

2. Infancy and Childhood:
   Pregnancy of mother. Birth complications. Nature of infantile and childhood diseases and injuries.

3. Schooling:
   Highest grade attained and at what age. Bright, normal or dull. Attitudes toward schoolmates and teachers.

4. Growth and Development:
   Disposition. Play life. Diversions. Sex life: Age when first manifested. Attitude toward own sex. Love affairs.

5. Personality:
   Degree of sociability and adaptability. Self-estimation. Leader or follower. Emotional stability. Antisocial trends. Dominant traits.

6. Occupation:
   Steadiness. Type and quality of work. Frequency of change of occupation.

7. Habits:
   Alcohol. Tobacco. Drugs.

8. Marital:
   Previous engagements. Divorces. Years married. Number of children. Compatibility and health of mate.

9. Home situation:

> Irritating factors. Special worries. Conduct toward other members of family. Response to authority or criticism.

10. Previous Attacks of Mental Illness:

> Age at onset. Nature of mental disease. Duration. Outcome.

11. Present Illness:

> Nature and time of onset. Apparent causes. Contributing factors. Further development of symptoms. Manner of treatment.

The Direct Examination

In substance the psychiatric examination of a patient is a friendly conference. It must not appear to be a brusque formality. A casual and sympathetic approach usually leads the patient to talk freely about his troubles and his experiences. It is not always the proper thing to take notes on significant observations, for some patients interpret this as a "test" and refuse to talk. Even though the examination may appear to be a haphazard conversation, the necessary material can be elicited and later organized to meet the requirements of a formal procedure. The best examination is one which provides for every humane consideration of the patient's feelings. Now and then the examiner should guide the patient by suggestion and by the proper tact will be able to bring out the more delicate and personal matters. The examiner's chief role is that of a good listener. The mere unburdening of worries and tensions becomes at once a part of the treatment in many instances.

Out of the material obtained from a patient who co-operates sufficiently and who is fairly accessible, the examiner can enter the findings under the following general topics:

a. **General appearance and behavior,** including a note as to dress, posture, expression of the face, the attitude toward the examiner and the nature of the patient's activity.

b. **Talk,** its general quality including some direct quotations; whether it is incoherent, rambling, groping, shows sudden suspension or the coining of meaningless words. The speed of conversation and the total amount of talk are equally important.

c. **Mood,** or the dominant emotional state of the patient. Note whether the patient is unduly happy, depressed, anxious, resentful, or excited, or whether he seems to be indifferent and shows notable lack of normal feeling.

d. **Content of Thought.**—Under this topic should be noted such elements as dominant ideas, superstitions, special religious beliefs, the content of dreams, illusions, delusions, and hallucinations.

e. **Orientation.**—It is important to determine whether the patient is aware of his immediate surroundings and knows where he is (spatial orientation), knows the date and the time of the year (temporal orientation), and is able to identify friends and relatives (personal orientation). Defects in orientation are common in old age and in advanced organic brain disease.

f. **Memory.**—The examiner can determine this by asking the patient for the year of birth or the date of marriage or by making inquiries about important events which occurred in the patient's early life. In older people it is necessary to determine whether there is a fairly good recollection of recent events such as those of yesterday or of the day before.

g. **Retention and Recall.**—This mental feature can be tested by giving the patient a number or a formula, preferably one which is not familiar or commonly used and asking him to repeat it. Or the patient can be given oral instructions to perform a succession of simple acts, and the failure or success of the performance will indicate the capacity to retain and to react to such instructions.

h. **General Intelligence.**—The intellectual capacity of the patient can be roughly estimated by his use of grammar, the wealth of his vocabulary, and the nature of his responses to questions pertaining to current events, history, geography, etc.

i. **Judgment and Insight.**—These highest qualities of mentality can be tested by asking the patient to express his opinion on political, social, or religious matters or to give a definition for such abstract terms as charity, reverence, or dishonesty. Insight can best be evaluated by inquiring of the patient whether he appreciates the nature of his illness and whether he is in need of treatment.

Naturally many patients, in spite of tact and careful handling, remain resistive to an interview or are evasive and cautious and frequently ignore the questions completely and become mute. The patient may be too depressed to converse with the examiner or too preoccupied with his own inner mental experiences to be able to answer questions. Finally a state of delirium or stupor may prevent any investigation of the mental status at the time. In such cases every objective note which can be made by physician and nurse becomes increasingly important in contributing toward an understanding of the mental disturbance. The facial expression, the posture, and any characteristic movements or unusual emotional manifestations become all-important elements in the record. Since the nurse is more frequently in contact with the patient than is the physician, the responsibility assigned to her to observe spontaneous conduct is not to·be minimized.

Special Mental Tests

The Rorschach Test.—Within the last twenty years, the Rorschach test has become widely accepted as a method of objectively evaluating personality structure and deviations. It is a test which purports the measurement of the more qualitative, nonintellectual traits of personality. Ten standard cards (ink blots) are presented to the patient in succession and he is asked informally to describe what he sees. In scoring, it is determined first whether the whole or certain portions of the ink blot elicited a response, secondly whether it was the form, color, shading, etc., which determined the patient's answer, and finally, what objects were formed in the otherwise meaningless shapes.

The intelligence, cultural background, thought content, degree of maturity or immaturity, degree of emotionality, degree of contact with reality can be determined from these answers. The test is used to differentiate the borderline psychotic from the psychoneurotic, the hysteria from the "organic" defect, the feebleminded from the constricted individual.not using all of the innate intelligence.

The Minnesota Multiphasic Personality Inventory.— This inventory is a psychological test designed to provide, in a single interview, scores on all the more important traits of personality.

The instrument itself consists of 550 questions covering a wide range of personality traits which the individual is asked to sort into three categories as they apply to him. The answers are indicated by index cards, "True," "False," and "Cannot say."

The personality characteristics now in available form for scoring are hypochondriasis, depression, hysteria, psychopathic personality, masculinity-femininity, paranoia, psychasthenia, schizophrenia and hypomania.

The Neurological Examination

The neurological examination is an essential part of every psychiatric case study, for many of the common mental diseases are associated with disturbances in the reflexes, with abnormal motor reactions, with paralysis, rigidity, spasticity and a wide range of other organic defects in the central nervous system.

The nurse cooperates in this portion of the examination by being at hand with a tray containing the necessary paraphernalia which should consist of the following: rubber reflex hammer, several small flashlights, one or two camel's hair brushes, one test tube to be filled with hot water and corked, another with cold water, an ophthalmoscope, and perhaps an instrument for measuring the strength of the grip—a dynamometer.

The General Physical Examination

It is almost needless to say that, like every person who is ill, the patient with mental disease must be thoroughly examined for any systemic or focal disease in organs and tissues other than those of the central nervous system. There are a fairly large number of general diseases which may injure the mental functions sufficiently to cause a psychosis.

Special Laboratory and Technical Examinations

There are many procedures and special tests which are indicated by the findings made in the clinical examination. A few should be mentioned because they are frequently indispensable in establishing a diagnosis and directing the therapy. Blood Wassermann and Kahn tests, spinal fluid studies, x-rays of the skull, chemical examination of the blood are examples of laboratory aids in the study of psychiatric problems. In suspected organic brain lesions such as brain tumors, the substitution of air for spinal fluid (encephalography and ventriculography) followed by x-ray studies has made possible the early recognition and treatment of these diseases. Even more recent are diagnostic devices such as the injection of radiopaque substances into the blood vessels (angiography) and the ingenious electro-encephalogram or "brain-wave" recorder, both of which find a useful application in neurology and psychiatry.

Electroencephalography

Electroencephalography is the recording of minute electric currents that accompany the activity of the brain.

These small currents or potential changes are amplified about a million times by an instrument somewhat similar to a radio amplifying set. It builds up the small currents to a voltage which will move a stylus or pen which records on a paper fed through the apparatus at a constant speed.

The nurse may assist in the preparation of the patient by helping in the placement of the electrodes on the patient's head. The electrodes are small lead discs which are applied to the scalp in various positions with a small amount of salt paste beneath each electrode. The electrodes are then cemented to the scalp by collodion which can be rapidly dried by a common hair drier. (Fig. 3) The electrode is connected by a fine

gauge copper wire to the control box of the electroencephalograph. The scalp requires no special preparation and the hair does not interfere with the placing
of the electrodes.

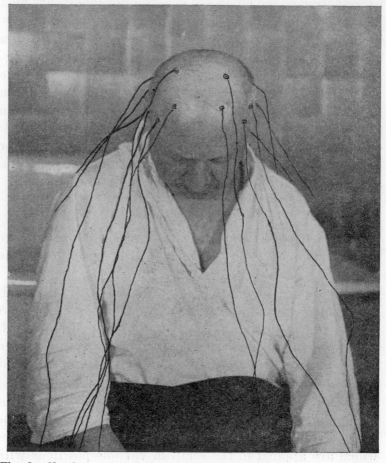

Fig. 3.—Showing one method of placing the electrodes on the scalp for
recording brain waves.

Although there may be slight variations in what are
considered to be normal records, there usualy is a definite regularity in the frequency and amplitude of the

brain waves. These normal waves, called alpha waves, have a frequency of 9 to 11 per second and an amplitude of from 10 to 50 microvolts (millionth of a volt). These waves are best studied in the occipital region with the patient at rest and with his eyes closed, but not asleep. About 90 per cent of the general population will show a record regarded as being within the limits of normal; 10 per cent will have a record which is either questionably normal or definitely abnormal.

Electroencephalography has proved of value in studying the epilepsies. Even in the interval between attacks, the record usually will show some variation in frequency, sometimes spoken of as a dysrhythmia, abnormal amplitude, or abnormal wave forms. During a clinical seizure, there is literally an electrical storm in the brain, and this produces definite changes in the electroencephalogram. In grand mal attacks, there is usually a discharge of fast, spike-like waves, and in petit mal seizures, there are large slow waves, about three per second, which at times alternate with a rapid spike-like wave.

Electroencephalography has also been useful in the localization of gross lesions of the cortex, such as brain tumors, and in the study of other organic brain diseases. It is being used in the investigation of the psychoses and personality disorders; however, its value in these conditions has not yet been established.

References

Bochner, Ruth, and Halpern, Florence: The Clinical Application of the Rorschach Test, New York, 1942, Grune & Stratton, Inc.

Franz, S. I.: Handbook of Mental Examination Methods, New York, 1919, The Macmillan Co.

Gibbs, Frederic A., and Gibbs, Erna L.: Atlas of Electroencephalography, Cambridge, Mass., 1941, Lew A. Cummings Co.

Hathaway, Starke R., and McKinley, Charnley I.: The Minnesota Multiphasic Personality Inventory, Minneapolis, 1943, University of Minnesota Press.

Hertz, Marguerite: Rorschach Bibliography, Cleveland, 1942, Brush
        Foundation Publication.
Kirby, George H.:   Guides for History Taking and Clinical Examination
        of Psychiatric Cases, Utica, N. Y., 1921, State Hospitals Press.
Preu, Paul: Outline of Psychiatric Case Study, New York, 1939, Paul
        B. Hoeber, Inc.
Rorschach, Hermann: Psychodiagnostics, New York, 1942, Grune & Strat-
        ton, Inc.
Wimmer, August: Psychiatric-Neurologic Examination Methods, trans-
        lated by Andrew W. Horsholt, St. Louis, 1919, The C. V. Mosby
        Company.

Questions for Chapter VI

The Examination of the Mental Patient

1. Why is it necessary to study every remote phase of an individual's life history?

2. There are three major parts to the complete examination of a mental patient. What are they?

3. From what sources may information regarding the patient's history be obtained? Is such information always reliable?

4. Enumerate the topics in the outline to be followed when compiling the life history of the patient.

5. Discuss the doctor's approach to the patient at the time of the psychiatric examination. What are his objectives?

6. Review the general outline used by the psychiatrist in his "direct examination" of the patient.

7. Name two special mental tests and indicate their particular value in the appraisal of the patient's personality.

8. Name several nervous system defects which may be among the findings of a neurological examination. List the articles required for the neurological examination.

9. Is the physical examination of great importance? Why?

10. Name four special laboratory tests frequently used in establishing a diagnosis. Name three technical examinations which are frequently used.

11. In stuporous or confused patients what important observations can be made by the nurse which become a significant part of the examination?

12. How may the nurse assist in preparing a patient for electroencephalography? What does the instrument record and in what conditions are the findings a valuable diagnostic aid?

CHAPTER VII

THE MANAGEMENT AND OBSERVATION OF THE MENTAL PATIENT

Adequate observation of a patient with mental disease represents the final and most complete method of examination. Under the eye of the experienced physician and the trained nurse in a hospital equipped and appointed for such a service, the behavior of the patient usually discloses those defects of mind and body which are the true basis of the psychic illness.

It is here that the psychiatric nurse can demonstrate her greatest value not only in properly guiding and treating her charges but in recording the necessary data which contribute toward establishing a correct diagnosis and prognosis. It matters not whether the patient be at home, in a general hospital, or in a special psychiatric institution, but it does matter a great deal as to whether the nurse in charge is trained to observe, record and interpret the important elements in the patient's behavior and to know how to meet the peculiar emergencies which arise in the management of the individual with a psychosis.

The Newly Admitted Patient

Perhaps in no other situation is a good first impression so important as it is in dealing with the mental patient who has just been admitted to the hospital. Every new patient is fearful of the traditional atmosphere associated with hospitals for mental disease, and many of them are influenced to come by misleading statements and promises. A kind word at the critical moment and an expression of interested sympathy from the ward

73

nurse may do more than anything else to determine the
patient's subsequent behavior. All preliminary procedures should be carefully and simply outlined to the
patient to allay suspicion and apprehension. A nurse's
uniform, a pleasant face, and an unperturbed tone of
voice are often the first step in successful mental therapy.

The bath and shampoo on admission furnish an excellent opportunity for the nurse to observe the body
for evidence of bruises, rash, deformities, and abdominal
distention. These must be carefully described in the
nurse's preliminary notes. It is advisable to withhold
artificial teeth and glasses from the patient until the
physician specifies whether or not these may be returned.
The nurse should remember to examine the mouth for
concealed drugs or valuables. The patient's clothing
can be carefully inspected for any material which may
furnish additional information as to the patient's habits
or peculiarities. All articles such as knives, pins,
razors, scissors, nail files, etc., must be locked up with other
fountain pens valuables. An accurate listing of all the patient's
clothing and property must be made on appropriate
forms. Shoes with hard soles or heels are to be replaced
by slippers if it is evident that the patient is greatly disturbed. In fact, any hard or metallic object, no matter
how small, which could possibly be turned to destructive
purposes must not be allowed to remain on the person.

Patients who are cooperative may be introduced to
the ward personnel and to other patients, taken to the
recreation room, and made to feel that the institution
can, with limitations, have the same informality in its
routine as one experiences at home. As much as possible, urge the new patient to talk in order that to some
degree the nature of the mental content can be ascertained and suitable precautions put into effect.

never leave pt. in restraints over six hrs. Bathe and massage

Violent and resistive patients may be secluded for a short period. Frequently the disturbed behavior is merely a temporary reaction to the new environment or is an expression of fear and resentment and subsides quickly.

The Supervision of the Mental Patient

One cannot demand a near-angelic disposition in every psychiatric nurse, but a well-balanced temperament is absolutely necessary. An intuitive capacity to sense the mood and attitude of her charges is a great asset; the ability to exhibit kindness and patience is indispensable.

The psychiatric nurse must at all times command the respect of the patient. Arguments are to be avoided; nor should threats of any kind be used as a method of controlling the turbulent patient. Appealing to a sense of humor, to honor, and to the better judgment will usually calm any but the very badly demented or extremely agitated individuals. Persuasion remains as effective a tool in controlling the psychiatric ward as it does in the schoolroom or the playground. Ridicule or any other form of denunciation cannot be tolerated. Thoughtless remarks about the sick person are to be condemned, for one must never forget that every patient who is not completely stuporous may be aware of everything which is said or done about him.

No matter how lowly the social station, the patient should be addressed by the surname, as Mr. Smith or Mrs. Brown. The use of the given name such as John or Mary is particularly resented by older people, for it implies a patronizing attitude and gives the patient the feeling that his relationship to the professional and nursing staff is that of a child.

Patients should be allowed to talk freely. It is well to be a good listener and to make mental notes of significant statements which should be entered at a later time on the patient's chart. A conversation with the patient carried on in a casual, conventional style, neither too formal nor too chatty, is best so that the patient is never made aware that he is being studied or tested. Some of the best material can be gathered by "listening in" on a conversation between a number of patients, for it is here that the individual is more genuine and spontaneous and is more likely to reveal his true mental behavior.

Management of the Disturbed Patient

Violent behavior in a psychotic patient is frequently an episode of short duration comparable to an emotional outburst in a normal person. It is true that in some psychoses, such as mania and the catatonic excitement of schizophrenia, the patient may be overactive, combative, and destructive for long periods, but at irregular intervals normal behavior may be observed. Excitement is usually short-lived and should be regarded as an immediate problem when it does occur.

Difficult though it may be, the cardinal rule in approaching a disturbed patient is to show no fear. Any evidence of panic on the part of the nurse will only serve to increase the patient's aggressive reactions.

No attempts should be made at physical control of a patient until it is evident that no amount of persuasion will do any good. If the patient has armed himself with some object such as a piece of glass, a curtain rod, or a broom, it may be advisable to request an attendant to approach the excited person from behind, envelop him with a blanket, and then obtain possession of the offending weapon. If it becomes necessary to carry out an order for mechanical restraint or emergency medication, the nurse must approach the patient with great caution, without a menacing attitude and only when assistants have been instructed to stand in readiness behind and to each side of the patient. Unless the excitement is extreme, the patient often subsides when he notes that he is about to be outmaneuvered. If necessary, he should be secured from behind by the wrists and shoulders and conducted to a secluded room. It is more rational to allow the free discharge of excitement by placing the patient in an empty room where he can pace back and forth than to adopt the habit of quelling each period of violence with hypnotics. The cold wet sheet pack or the continuous tub offers a safe method of abating the excitement and controlling the patient.

If medication by mouth is necessary in a resistive or excited patient, a desirable method is to place the patient in a chair, with an assistant holding the arms behind the back of the chair; then, with the head slightly extended and anchored by holding the chin, the medicine can be usually administered without additional difficulty. If the teeth are clenched, never resort to the practice of closing the nostrils. This is a dangerous and vicious maneuver, particularly in elderly patients or those who have cardiovascular disease. Far more preferable is to request the physician for another method of administration, such as hypodermic medication or an intravenous injection of an appropriate sedative.

Restraint

This term usually is applied to mechanical methods of controlling excited patients, although it must not be forgotten that sedatives and hypnotics are also essentially forms of restraint. Mechanical restraint is that which limits activity by the use of sheets, canvas jackets, straps, cuffs, or heavy blankets.

In general, modern psychiatry looks upon simple mechanical restraint with disfavor. As a last resort it

can be applied to patients who are likely to injure themselves and to delirious and confused subjects who may
fall out of bed and sustain a skull fracture. Restraint
may be used when it is necessary to tube-feed a very
resistive patient. In every instance where mechanical
restraint is indicated, it must be applied only on direct
order of the physician in charge.

General Hygiene on Mental Wards

The proper ventilation of a psychiatric ward is an all-
important item, and it must be continually maintained to
avoid the well-known "institutional odor." The windows should be opened sufficiently to allow free movement of air, but draughts must be avoided, for mental
patients require a warm room because many of them are
ambulatory and wear light clothing. Bedclothing must
be adequate and warm.

Cleanliness is of prime importance; the mouth and
teeth should be cleansed at least twice a day to avoid infections and halitosis.

When cleansing tub baths are ordered, the procedure
must be closely supervised. An attendant should prepare the bath before the patient enters the room, and
the patient should never be left alone. The drain should
be removed before the patient steps out of the tub. The
attendant should submit a report of bruises or any evidence of skin eruption or laceration.

Elimination

It is essential that mental patients have proper and
regular elimination. The nurse must so instruct the
ward personnel that distended bladders and rectal impactions do not occur. The average mental patient who
is ambulatory can be trained quickly to understand the

importance of reporting the frequency of elimination and any other unusual feature in this necessary function. Bed patients are easily observed in this respect. Frequent inspection of the abdomen in confused and stuporous individuals is necessary to prevent distention of the bladder and fecal impaction. If there is a definite retention of urine, placing the patient in a tepid bath may be effective in inducing urination. Otherwise catheterization is indicated.

The nurse must proceed with extreme care in catheterizing a disturbed patient, never using anything but a soft rubber tube. The upper part of the body is immobilized by a restraining sheet wrapped around the arms and across the chest. The legs should be held by two assistants. The catheter should be sterile and the hands scrupulously clean. The instrument should be inserted slowly and with great patience, for there is danger of trauma to the urethra and bladder.

The same care and precautions are demanded if an enema is to be administered. The technique is otherwise that which is applied to any patient who requires this aid to normal evacuation of the bowels. Colonic irrigation may be supplemented in badly constipated patients. The procedure is described in the chapter on hydrotherapy.

Nutrition

Mentally ill patients often refuse to eat for many and varied reasons. It is well to ascertain just what reason the patient proffers for refusal to eat.

The proper tact and ingenuity in persuading the patient to eat are usually successful except in severe catatonic block or melancholia. Some patients refuse food because they have hallucinations, the voices telling them not to eat. At intervals when the hallucinated condition is not present, such patients are capable of taking food. Patients who are depressed may feel that they are unworthy of food or state that they are too poor to pay for the meal. Consequently when asked to help in the ward work this objection is nullified, or they may be shown that the food is wasted if they do not consume it. Those who believe that the food is poisoned are extremely unreasonable, but they may eat if allowed to prepare their own food or serve it themselves from the food cart. Occasionally the paranoid patient will willingly eat from a tray which has been prepared for another patient. Canned foods, eggs in the shell or potatoes in jackets are selected frequently because these do not lend themselves, according to the patient's reasoning, to contamination. A patient may eat food sent in or prepared by relatives, and no other. If relatives are willing to cooperate, this arrangement is preferred to forced feeding.

Untidy patients should be spoon fed in seclusion, but the nurse should make every attempt to teach such patients to feed themselves. Some patients eat too much and require careful watching at meal times in order that they do not gorge themselves or deprive others of their food.

All trays can be prepared attractively with small portions, the nurse allowing second helpings if such are indicated.

If forced feeding is necessary, exceeding care is to be taken to avoid bruising the patient's lips or tongue. An enamel feeding cup with the spout protected by rubber tubing may be used to give fluids. Spoon-feeding should always be a slow and patient procedure, to allow the patient ample time to swallow and to make sure that the food is not accumulated in the buccal cavities or the pharynx. When forced feedings are unsuccessful, the physician should be notified and the patient placed on the tube-feeding list.

Those patients whose weekly weight chart shows loss should be given extra nourishment between meals.

The nurse's attempts to make the meal hour attractive will be well repaid. Trays and dining rooms may be neat and colorful. Quietness should prevail, and untidy patients should not be allowed in the dining room. If the nurse learns her patient's likes and dislikes regarding certain food, meal times will be less trying to both patient and nurse.

Procedure for Tube Feeding

A tube feeding can be given easily with the patient in a comfortable position if he sits in a chair. However, if the patient is resistive, and many of them are, the feeding may be given with the patient in bed. At times he will need to be mummied in a blanket, or if he is very resistive, restrained during the procedure. Have the patient and the bed well protected with rubber sheeting and a towel.

The tray should contain a cold stomach or nasal feeding tube. It may be cooled by placing it in the refrigerator for a short time before the feeding is given, or it may be placed on cracked ice. A lubricating agent such as glycerine or mineral oil is supplied, and a large kidney basin should be at hand. If a stomach tube is used, a mouth gag may be necessary. The feeding, warmed to 105° F., may consist of rich eggnog or any formula which the doctor orders.

Before feeding, the patient should be offered food. If he refuses, the procedure is carried out, the doctor inserting the tube. If medication is given, it should be poured in first. The amount of the feeding will be ordered by the doctor and will vary according to necessity. Water is sometimes given in addition to the feeding. The fluid should be poured slowly but constantly so that no air enters with the feeding. Great care should be taken when withdrawing the tube that all fluid has run out. Pinch the tube so that any fluid adhering to the tube will not run out into the patient's lungs. Lung abscess may result if this happens.

Some patients try to regurgitate their feedings. Such patients should be restrained before feeding and left in restraint from one-half to three-quarters of an hour after the feeding.

The tubing should be cleaned immediately after use, as the eggnog will dry in the tube otherwise, and it is almost impossible to clean if this happens.

Regulating Sleep

Insomnia is a common feature of many mental disorders, and, in addition, the sleepless patient may create considerable disturbance at night. A confidential discussion of the fears and worries with the nurse and a word or two of assurance from her are often more effective than a sedative tablet.

Patients sleep better if a moderate amount of exercise is provided for during the day. Physical exertion or mental excitement just before bedtime should be discouraged. A hot drink or a very light lunch at bedtime may induce restful sleep. A cool, well-ventilated room, a hot-water bottle to the feet and subdued lighting are the usual prerequisites to sleep.

Some patients feign sleep, others sleep fitfully, still others may awake early in the morning hours. There is no fixed rule as to what constitutes normal sleep, but a patient who is restless and wakeful for many nights is undoubtedly suffering with insomnia, and some supporting medication may be given.

Too frequently there is a tendency to obtain routine orders for sedative medication in insomnia, and the drug is given for an indefinite time without special study of the patient's response to such perfunctory treatment. Occasional sedatives may be necessary, but they should be varied in kind and discontinued after a short time. It is the duty of the physician to dictate the type and amount of sedation, and the responsibility of the nurse to observe and report the reaction to such medication. Good nursing and medical care on a mental ward is inversely proportional to the amount of sedatives and hypnotics which are administered for sleeplessness.

Precautions Against Self-Injury and Suicide

In mental disease normal sensibility to pain may be distorted, and patients may injure themselves without showing signs of pain or discomfort. It is necessary to protect them from hot radiators, and, when hot-water bottles are applied, the skin is to be frequently inspected for burns. If mental patients are encased in plaster splints, the same unceasing scrutiny of the skin and the circulation must be made to avoid abrasions, infection, or gangrene.

Psychotic patients may harm themselves by many unpredictable methods, the reason for this being some impulsion or motive arising out of a hallucinated state. Patients have been known to swallow pins, nails, rings, pieces of bedspring or even spoons—not with the idea of suicide but because of a peculiar perversion of taste. Occasionally a schizophrenic individual has the distorted desire to push pins, needles, and nails into the skin or the scalp.

Suicide is an ever-present potentiality in the psychotic patient, particularly in the depressed individual. Experience furnishes no safe rule whereby the impulse can be accurately predicted. The impulse to self-destruction may appear without warning, and again the patient may carry out a carefully premeditated plan to end his own life.

The nurse does well to acquaint herself with the ways and means of patients with suicidal intent. Patients attempt to drown themselves in bath tubs, to hang themselves with belts, sheets, neckties, towels, and bathrobe cords. They cut their wrists with glassware, watch crystals, eyeglasses, bits of windowpane, and safety razor blades. They may seize bottles of antiseptic solution from dressing trays or obtain cleaning solution from a utility room and swallow the fluid in an instant. Jumping from a window sill or from the head of the bed to the floor head first is a method utilized by severely agitated or depressed individuals.

Chewing and swallowing a thermometer occurs frequently enough to become a problem of great import when it is essential to record daily temperatures. Running in front of, and deliberately falling before, a passing automobile, and jumping from a balcony are examples of self-destruction by a patient who is allowed to go outdoors without close supervision.

Patients who show by word or action that they are potentially suicidal are placed on "suicidal observation." All depressed individuals should be so classified without exception. If the previous history contains any hint of self-destructive impulse or attempted suicide, this is also an indication for caution. There is no basis for the belief that individuals who talk about suicide rarely take their own lives; they require the same close supervision as those who do not make the threat.

All the patients on the "suicidal list" must be under constant scrutiny. Asleep or awake, while eating, dressing or bathing, or at toilet, the patient should be under the watchful eye of an attendant or nurse. The clothing, the bed, and the entire room should be searched daily for any objects which may be turned to self-destructive purposes. Periodic observation during the hours of sleep— in short a constant vigilance—is the rule in all cases where suicide is even a remote possibility.

Accidents

Many distressing and unavoidable accidents occur on the wards of mental hospitals for obvious reasons. Most of these are the direct result of the disturbed behavior of the patient. Altercations between patients are probably the most frequent occasions for trouble. More active patients jostle the infirm and those whose muscular coordination is poor. Falls from bed, sudden collapse, convulsions, burns, and fractures, particularly in elderly people, are critical emergencies which the nurse should be prepared to meet in the routine management of a psychiatric ward. Patients may injure themselves by breaking glass panes in attempting to escape. The nurse should bear in mind that a certain percentage of her charges are continually plotting escape—a not infrequent occurrence in even the best managed institutions.

All accidents or unusual emergencies which occur should be reported in detail on the nurse's record and, not only should the physician be notified, but an accurate description of the accident in writing should be submitted to the administrative officer who in turn can notify the interested relatives.

Systematic Observation of the Patient's Behavior

Probably no method of recording data on the behavior of mental patients is better than a complete recital of one's own experience with the individual, with direct quotations from his conversation and a simple account of his conduct in everyday language. However, like many other phenomena, abnormal behavior can be recorded in a standardized or systematic fashion by the use of various set forms or charts which can be interpreted by more than one individual and which can demonstrate certain trends or major elements in behavior.

Most ingenious and practical is the *behavior chart* devised by Dr. Adolph Meyer for the Henry Phipps Psychiatric Clinic at Johns Hopkins Hospital. It has met with great favor, is widely used, and is generally known as the "Johns Hopkins Behavior Sheet."

Fig. 4 is a reproduction of a greatly modified form of Meyer's behavior chart. In the extreme left portion of this form is a list of the most common features which may be found to exist in the behavior of a mentally ill individual. These are arranged in a significant order. The graphic portion of the chart allows for a recording of each feature for each day of the month. If during a given day a given symptom is prominently and consistently present, this can be recorded by a complete cross. If this particular feature is manifested only during a part of the day, the entry should be a simple oblique line or half a cross; if the symptom is demonstrated only at irregular or infrequent intervals, a quarter cross or one-half an oblique line will show this graphically.

It will be noted that a portion of the behavior features in the middle zone of the chart is separated from the rest by two double lines. These features are grouped in this

Abulia — lack of will power
Echolalia - senseless repetition of words.
Echopraxia - senseless repetition of acts

manner because they, and no others, will be found to be present if a normal or nonpsychotic patient is under observation. Hence the normal zone in the chart is a

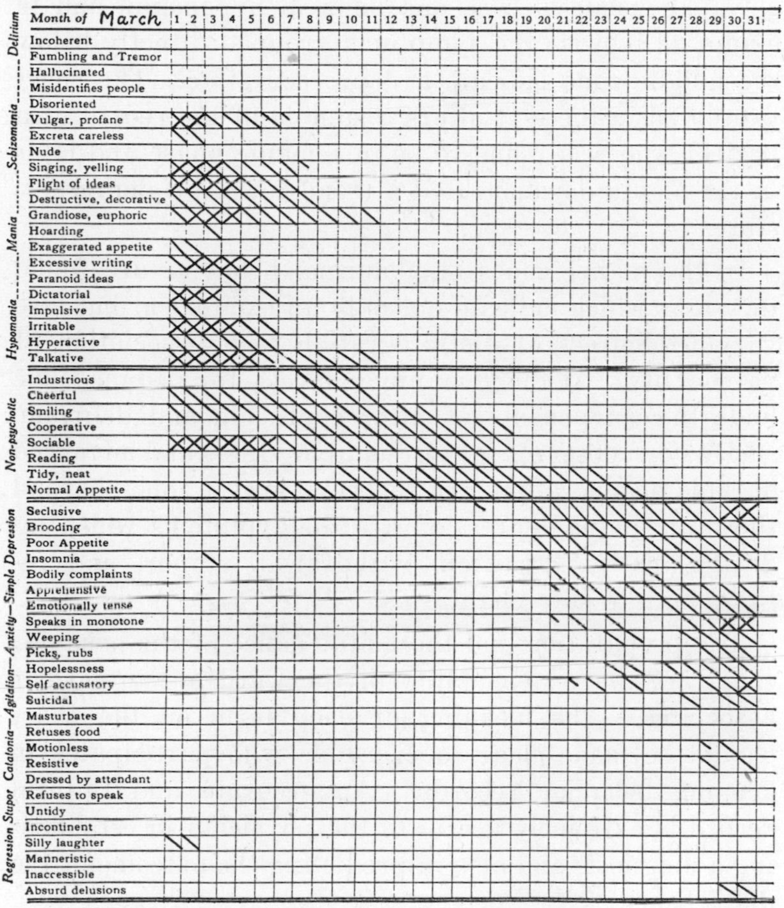
Month of March
1 2 3 4 5 6 7 8 9 10 11 12 13 14 15 16 17 18 19 20 21 22 23 24 25 26 27 28 29 30 31
Delirium
Incoherent
Fumbling and Tremor
Hallucinated
Misidentifies people
Disoriented
Schizomania
Vulgar, profane
Excreta careless
Nude
Singing, yelling
Flight of ideas
Mania
Destructive, decorative
Grandiose, euphoric
Hoarding
Exaggerated appetite
Excessive writing
Paranoid ideas
Hypomania
Dictatorial
Impulsive
Irritable
Hyperactive
Talkative
Non-psychotic
Industrious
Cheerful
Smiling
Cooperative
Sociable
Reading
Tidy, neat
Normal Appetite
Simple Depression
Seclusive
Brooding
Poor Appetite
Insomnia
Bodily complaints
Anxiety
Apprehensive
Emotionally tense
Speaks in monotone
Weeping
Agitation
Picks, rubs
Hopelessness
Self accusatory
Suicidal
Catatonia
Masturbates
Refuses food
Motionless
Resistive
Stupor
Dressed by attendant
Refuses to speak
Untidy
Regression
Incontinent
Silly laughter
Manneristic
Inaccessible
Absurd delusions

Fig. 4.—Behavior sheet modified from the Johns Hopkins Chart. The recorded data reveals a manic excitement in the first half of the month and a depressed phase in the latter part.

middle band, and deviations from the normal will be recorded by positive recordings above and below this zone.

A close study of the behavior symptoms just above the normal zone will show that these are features which generally develop in a person with an excited state or elevated mood, such as one finds in hypomania and in mania. Likewise the symptoms grouped directly below the middle zone indicate a depressed state. The chart presented in the text offers a sample of the record of a patient who was found to be in a manic phase and later in the month demonstrated a trend toward a depressive state.

In the higher zones of abnormal behavior are found the signs which indicate not only an excitement but also varying degrees of distintegration and dissociation of personality. At the very upper levels, for instance, one finds the components of utter confusion and delirium, such as one observes in serious toxic states and advanced organic degeneration. In the very lowest zones beyond those of simple depression are the symptoms which indicate apathy, dejection, withdrawal, stupor, and regression into silly phantasies.

The preparation and the maintenance of the behavior chart are the responsibility of the ward nurse and her associates. The meaning of each term on the chart should be made clear to everyone who participates in keeping behavior records. An accurate and faithful record is extremely useful to the physician in establishing a diagnosis and also in predicting the outcome of the disturbance.

Most of the terms used in the behavior chart are self-explanatory, and it would be better that every term were so simple that it could not be readily misunderstood. However, a few are somewhat technical and require a little elaboration.

Incoherent: Conversation is rambling; ideas are not naturally related.

Fumbling and Tremor: Purposeless picking with the fingers. Shaking of the hands during voluntary movement or during rest.

Hallucinated: A false perception through sight, hearing, smelling or tasting. Unless the patient talks freely of such false perceptions or concedes them when questioned, it is not advisable to note that this symptom exists, even though the behavior and attitude may lead one to suspect that hallucinosis is present.

Misidentifies People: The patient calls the nurse, physician, or other patients by strange names or assigns different identities to his own friends and relatives.

Disoriented: An inability to know the time or date; gets lost on the ward; cannot locate his own bed; fails to recognize his own relatives.

Vulgar, Profane: Coarse talk, crude behavior; swears, uses vile language.

Excreta Careless: Indifferent as to where and how bodily excretions, such as feces and expectoration, are left.

Flight of Ideas: A rapid shift from one idea to another in conversation, with much digression and distractibility.

Grandiose, Euphoric: Expressing ideas of great wealth or power; a feeling of elation.

Paranoid Ideas: The term is to be applied to false ideas which, however, have the quality of being believable; they should not be utterly absurd. For instance, if a patient claims that he has been "framed" by his relatives, or that other patients abuse him or that his friends cheated him in some financial deal, such would be good examples of "paranoid ideas."

Dictatorial: Making unreasonable demands; insisting on being obeyed; "bossy."

Emotionally Tense: Showing anxiety, inability to relax, restless, agitated, perplexed.

Manneristic: Given to peculiar poses, bodily attitudes or unusual facial grimacing. Repeating senseless movements.

Silly Laughter: Smiling or laughing for no appropriate reason.

Inaccessible: Impossible to determine the content of the patient's thinking. Living within one's own mental life. Another term which may be used here is *autism.*

Absurd Delusions: Under this symptom should be included all false ideas which are of an unbelievable nature, such as "The President of the United States controls my thoughts through radio." "I am here to save the patients from being destroyed by devils." Expressions of queer delusions are typical of badly disorganized personalities such as one sees in schizophrenia.

No behavior chart, no matter how adequately maintained, can possibly record all the outstanding features in the behavior of a psychotic patient. Detailed notes should always be made of an unusual episode or of any significant statement made by the patient. Whenever any question arises as to the proper method of recording certain characteristics, the physician should be consulted. It is the physician who makes the interpretations in the final analysis. Much of his success in diagnosis and treatment depends on how conscientiously the psychiatric nurse keeps her behavior sheets.

References

Bennett, Abram K., and Purdy, Avis B.: Psychiatric Nursing Technic, Philadelphia, 1940, F. A. Davis Co.
Ebaugh, Franklin G.: The Care of the Psychiatric Patient in General Hospitals, Chicago, 1940, American Hospital Association.

Ingram, Madelene E.: Principles of Psychiatric Nursing, Philadelphia, 1942, W. B. Saunders Co.
Sadler, William S.: Psychiatric Nursing, St. Louis, 1937, The C. V. Mosby Company.
White, William Allen: Outlines of Psychiatry, ed. 9, New York, 1923, Nervous & Mental Disease Publishing Co.

Questions on Chapter VII

The Management and Observation of the Mental Patient

1. With what skills may the psychiatric nurse demonstrate her greatest value?
2. Discuss the nurse's attitude and approach to the newly admitted patient.
3. What data must the nurse's notes contain concerning the new patient?
4. Carefully outline the care of the patient's property upon admission. What is done with artificial teeth, glasses, valuables, harmful objects, and clothing?
5. Give some good reasons why the nurse should attempt to establish a friendly relationship with the patient.
6. Make a written list of the necessary qualities of the good psychiatric nurse. Make another list of some of the things a good psychiatric nurse would never do.
7. What is the cardinal rule in approaching a disturbed patient?
8. Under what conditions is it permissible to make attempts at physical control of an excited patient?
9. Be prepared to demonstrate the proper physical approach to a disturbed patient. What preliminary plans should be made before approaching such a patient?
10. Discuss the following factors in the regulation of sleep: fears and worries of the patient, exercise before bedtime, ventilation of the patient's room, lighting, precautions in the administration of a sedative.
11. List the methods of self-injury which a patient may employ. In each instance discuss the preventive measures which must be taken.
12. Discuss the behavior chart as to the following points: purpose, method of recording symptoms on the behavior sheet and the nurse's notes, and the responsibility of the nurse in keeping these records.
13. Define ten terms found on the behavior sheet which are not self-explanatory.

CHAPTER VIII

AFFECTIVE REACTION TYPES—THE MANIC-DEPRESSIVE PSYCHOSES

There are individuals who by innate temperament have an unusual vivacity, indulge in a wide range of activity, and have a quick and appropriate response to every situation. They make friends easily and have a facile ease in expressing their feelings, which may be at one time those of elation and again those of moodiness and dejection. They are possessed of floods of energy which for a time seem inexhaustible but this overactivity may be interrupted by periods of underactivity and inertia. Bleuler calls this the syntonic temperament, and Kretschmer refers to such normal people as cyclothymes. Because these people have frank, open personalities, a good intuitive knowledge of others, a good sense of humor, and an easy and natural manner, many of them attain a remarkable degree of success. Their aggressive nature and their capacity to apply themselves with unlimited enthusiasm when the occasion requires it make them the leaders in social movements, the organizers, executives, and the more colorful characters in politics, medicine, art, and in all the practical professions. What weaknesses the syntone may show in personality performances are due to his susceptibility to being carried away by his emotions, to indulgence in superficial thinking and activity, and to a disinclination to think in a cool, unimpassioned way. Syntones are also the sensual enjoyers of life, which trait is frequently exaggerated so that excesses may appear particularly in matters of drink, food, and love. In keeping with such tendencies, the syntone or cyclothyme tends to have a bulky, stocky body called by Kretschmer the pyknic constitution in which the vegetative function is so vigorous that there is a strong tendency to overweight.

Manic-depressive psychosis is a mental upset which springs out of such a temperament. It is characterized by a wide and sustained swing in mood, either in the direction of elation or of depression. One phase is frequently followed by the other. For a long time it was believed that mania was one disease and melancholia was another, but it can be readily shown that the same patient frequently suffers with both phases in alternate manner.

Etiology.—It is assumed that the basic cause is an inherited or innate tendency to hyperactive temperament. Sixty to 80 per cent of these patients have a family history with such trends. Occasionally there seems to be no exciting or precipitating cause, and the attack may arise from a clear sky. In such cases the disease is termed *constitutional* or *endogenous*. Many of the patients, however, disclose a fairly specific precipitating factor which may be a mental tension or a physical disease, and the mania or depression is then called *reactive*. Reactive psychoses generally have a better outlook than those which arise without any immediate provocation.

Symptoms of the Manic Phase.—The three outstanding symptoms are (a) elated mood, (b) overtalkativeness with flight of ideas, and (c) excessive psychomotor activity. The elated mood is so pronounced and sustained that the patient feels unusually well, has no great sense of repression, and has the feeling that every good thing is possible or will soon be consummated, every wish will be fulfilled. Ideas emerge in an easy, fluidlike manner; thinking seems to be effortless; memory is quickened;

and the patient shows a quick but superficial wit. There is a great sense of self-security; fears are pushed to the background; and the patient is overaggressive, cocksure

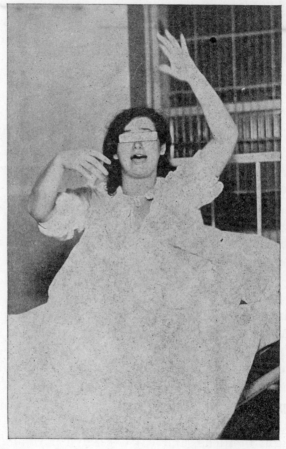

Fig. 5.—Acute mania, demonstrating great elation and psychomotor activity.

in his opinions, and ready to talk with conviction on anything and everything. The ego is unrestrained and ideas pour out so rapidly and with such ease that the tongue cannot give them full expression. Hence, the patient utters only segments of ideas and jumps from one to another in a rapid barrage. There is a quick appreciation of persons and objects, a smart-aleck appraisal of others, and a tendency to argument. The patient is domineering, will brook no restraint, and becomes irritable, denunciatory, and hypercritical of everything which interferes with his desire for free action. He becomes overactive, obtrusive, and extends this excessive motor excitement into every direction. Frequently when crossed or when denounced for his irritating behavior, he becomes noisy, belligerent, and violent. His insight is always poor. The manic's interest is in the outside world rather than in himself. His ideation is concerned with his environment; in fact, in acute mania the patient can almost be said to be at the mercy of his environment.

Types of Mania.—The symptoms given above are the features common to all forms of mania. There are other features which modify the picture and justify a loose subdivision which, however, is not clean-cut for one form may readily merge with another.

Hypomania

This is the mildest form of mania; yet a patient with hypomania may be a greater problem and nuisance than any other manic for the very reason that the layman may regard him as being merely a vivacious fellow who is being badly abused. For a time he is considered a quick and witty person who has many enthusiasms, many wonderful plans for the future and one with "personality plus." Very soon, however, he becomes interfering, domineering, and unable to keep to the subject at hand. He becomes intolerant of other opinions, ruthless in his denunciations and impatient with the "stupidity" and "sluggish" mentality of others. Many schemes are planned but only a few are started and none are finished. He has a glib reason for everything he does, concedes no mistakes, and rationalizes all his activities. He lacks moral restraint, may become coarse in his remarks, and may indulge in sexual and alcoholic excesses. He spends money recklessly and in a few weeks may impoverish his family and totally dissipate his estate.

When he is finally committed to a hospital—he never goes willingly—he becomes one of the most difficult patients to manage. Demands are made for immediate release, and the patient calls for an attorney and warns those in charge to be prepared for legal retaliation. He insists on proofs of insanity and is ready with a rebuttal to every charge made against him. He is continually busy doing something, particularly collecting clippings and writing letters to important officials outlining the abuses which he suffers. He accuses the physicians and nurses of immorality, of being connivers, and of running a vile institution. His memory is keen, his repartee is quick, and he relishes an argument with patients, nurses, and attendants. Rarely does he become confused or hallucinated, but his insight into his real condition is poor and his judgment is very bad.

To picture more clearly some of these clinical types a case of hypomania is presented as follows:

M. H., 48 years old, was a real estate salesman by occupation. His mother had a mental illness at 46 years of age which was probably a melancholia. He had been educated in private schools and earned a college degree in business administration. During his junior year (1921), he failed to win a particular scholarship and became morose, sleepless, and nervous for a period of two months. In 1925 he entered an auto sales contest and won first prize which was a trip to Havana. While on this trip he became moderately intoxicated and insisted on eating every meal at the captain's table where he told obscene stories and embarrassed the women passengers. He participated in frequent brawls with the stewards and complained to the purser on every occasion. On disembarking at New York, instead of returning to his home city, he remained there. He demanded the most pretentious accommodations at the hotel, and, when these were unavailable, the patient entered into a noisy altercation with the manager which resulted in his being sent to Bellevue Hospital. He remained there for three months and finally returned to his parents' home.

The present attack began about six weeks before admission. At that time he was engaged in selling real estate in a new subdivision. He became extremely active, arose early, and accosted prospective clients in street cars, waiting rooms, and hotel corridors. He talked in such convincing manner that he made a good record in the first week of the sale. Only a ten-dollar deposit was necessary to close a deal. The patient continued to send in many deposits, bragged about his sales ability, argued noisily with his fellow salesmen, and finally was arrested because he failed to pay the street car conductor for his transportation. He then entered a damage suit against the car company for $100,000. The attorney who was approached realized the absurdities of the patient's claims and filed the charges against the patient.

Immediately after admission he demanded to see the head physician and requested permission to use the telephone. He was fairly coherent but was circumstantial in his conversation. When asked a simple question, his reply was a long, rambling, and digressive account. After being continually reminded to answer the question pointedly, he did so, only to return to another long digression. He made unreasonable demands of the nurses and attendants and, if refused, he became abusive, sarcastic, and irritable. At this time it was discovered that when a client refused to pay $10 down on a lot, the patient would draw the sum out of his own bank account and forge a signature on the sales contract. This explained his amazing sales success.

He spent a great deal of his time writing letters to the mayor, to various attorneys, and influential citizens. He wrote these missives on odd pieces of paper with pencil and in a broad, sweeping hand, underlining almost every other word, and capitalizing others. Every day at ward rounds he met the physicians at the door and began to revile them. He particularly enjoyed arguing with the doctors, demanding any evidence proving that he was insane, and consistently denied all charges of misbehavior. In a loud voice he promised to have the hospital superintendent removed, the doctors exposed as quacks, and the orderlies jailed for beating him. He was suggestively lewd in his conversation with all the nurses, except a young pupil to whom he proposed marriage. When it was pointed out to him that he was already married, he harshly announced that he would divorce his wife because "she leaves me in this crazy dump."

Throughout ten weeks he remained on the disturbed ward, the constant center of commotion, a chronic critic of everything and everybody about him, consistently refusing all medication, collecting and hoarding papers, combs, magazines, and all sorts of trash, and acquiring many bruises in frequent affrays with other patients. Occasionally he was very agreeable and jolly, particularly if he was allowed to do all the talking. On these occasions he was fond of reciting cheap parodies of famous poems in a quick, witty fashion. Some of these he had not quoted since his high school days.

While he had the belief that he was wrongfully incarcerated and that he was being abused, he harbored no other delusional ideas, and at no time was he confused or hallucinated. His intellect was keen, his memory, particularly for trivial things, remarkable but he had no insight into his abnormal exaltation and irritability and his judgment was decidedly bad.

Acute Mania

Mania may develop very suddenly and give little or no warning symptoms. This is particularly true of the more violent forms, in which the signs of the disease may become full-blown overnight or within a few hours. Acute mania is very much like hypomania, but the condition is more intense. The elated mood is so pronounced that the patient is silly, laughs boisterously, and talks at the top of his voice with a wild flight of ideas, displays fits of anger and easily provoked irritability. There may be incoherence, some confusion, and disorientation with a tendency to misidentify people about him and to talk in a jargonlike manner to himself. Invariably the patient is obscene, destructive, and violent. Assaults upon other patients are frequent. The patient is con-

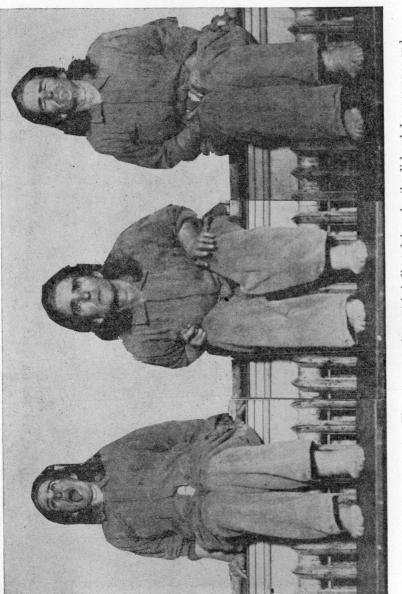

Fig. 6.—An acute mania. The extreme excitement is indicated here by the disheveled appearance and the facial grimacing.

tinually "on the go," walking for hours back and forth in his room, climbing to the window sill, spitting upon the walls, and banging on the panels of his door, demanding release. Again there may be short periods of good humor, some insight into his noisy behavior and even an apologetic attitude. The confusional features are mild; the irritable and elated mood is outstanding; and judgment is exceedingly poor. The following story is that of a typical acute mania.

A. G., a 38-year-old woman of German extraction whose father was a high-strung musician of great talents and at one time the director of a famous symphony orchestra. Her mother was a quiet, timid, almost unemotional type, but deeply religious and devoted to her family. The patient herself was somewhat strong-willed, spoiled in her girlhood, and given to temper tantrums even as late as her adolescence. At the age of 18 years she ran away to be married to her husband who was a stolid, home-loving type and who adjusted himself very well to her frequent moods and bad temper. She had three children, living and well, on whom she lavished a great deal of attention.

Three months before her admission two of the children had scarlet fever. Although a trained nurse was in attendance, the patient insisted on being at hand and as a result made herself a nuisance. She worried continually for three weeks during which the children were acutely ill; she slept very little, and developed marked tremor of the hands. The family physician was consulted and expressed the opinion that she had a mild nervous collapse and also that she might have goiter. The patient convinced herself that she had goiter and the very next day went to a shrine in an adjoining town to be cured of it by prayer. She prayed for several hours and at the end of that time became incoherent, noisy, and somewhat elated. The shrine attendants placed her in an ambulance which conveyed her to a large hospital clinic. There she manifested no clear signs of hyperthyroidism, but instead became noisy, talkative, and screamed so loudly that she was at once transferred to the psychopathic hospital.

On admission she slapped the nurse, addressed the house physician as God, made the sign of the cross, and laughed loudly when she was asked to don the hospital garb. This she promptly tore into shreds. She remained nude for several hours before she was restrained in bed. She sang at the top of her voice, screamed through the window, and leered at the patients promenading in the recreation yard. She was very untidy and incontinent, smearing her excreta about the floor and walls. Frequently she would utter the words, "God, Thou Holy One," cross herself, laugh, and then give vent to vile expletives while she carried out suggestive movements of the body. She yelled for water, and, when this was proffered, she threw the tin cup across the room.

For several weeks she remained in restraint in bed or was given continuous hydrotherapy. Tube feeding was necessary for two weeks after which she ate sparingly from her own tray. There were periods lasting one or two days when she was relatively quiet and would sit almost motionless upon a mattress in her own room. These short periods of apathy were soon followed by more excitement and violence. Her husband visited her frequently, but she rarely paid him much attention, and on several occasions called him a "despoiler" and pushed him from the room.

Two months after admission she was given metrazol treatment and had a series of five convulsions. For nine days she was practically normal so that her relatives were on the point of taking her home. However, she soon relapsed into her manic excitement. A week later she was given two more metrazol injections and promptly became normal again except that she was irritable and somewhat suspicious. Finally at the end of three months she was regarded as being recovered and was discharged.

Delirious Mania

Delirious mania is the highest degree of mania and may develop from a milder form, but more frequently appears suddenly and with very few warning signs. Although it cannot always be demonstrated, an infection, a drug intoxication or an injury to the head may be the factor causing the delirium which is added to the simple manic excitement.

The patient with delirious mania is definitely confused, has no appreciation of his surroundings, and may be hallucinated. There are much tremor and fumbling with the bedclothes, continuous excitement, screaming, singing, and incoherent yelling. Rarely can the patient answer the simplest questions.

M. V., a schoolteacher 31 years old, with a negative family history except for the fact that a younger brother was a chronic alcoholic. Ten days before admission she complained of a sore throat for which she was given sodium salicylate, but she took this medication for only four days. She complained later of pain in the right jaw. Two days before admission she became irritable, talkative, and insisted that she heard a man talking behind the bathroom door. She persisted in searching the room in question every few minutes. She was extremely restless and, when admonished, became noisy and combative. When put to bed, she was feverish and began to sing at the top of her voice. A physician who was called gave her an opiate, after which she slept for several hours. Early in the morning she resumed her noisy behavior and required restraint in bed.

On admission she was incoherent, ignored all questions except to cry out at intervals, "Keep going, keep going." She sat up in bed, picking continually at the bedclothes and tearing threads out of the counterpane. Her mouth was very dry; the lips were covered with sores; and her tongue was heavily coated. Her pulse rate was 110, and her temperature was 38.4° C. The right side of the jaw in the region of the parotid gland was moderately swollen. She was incontinent and soiled her bedclothing frequently. It was impossible to give her nourishment by spoon feeding, for she either clenched her teeth or spewed the food in all directions. Tube feeding was necessary for several days.

Her temperature dropped to normal on the twelfth hospital day and the parotid swelling subsided. She remained silly and showed a fondness for decorating herself with bread crusts, and painting her face with beet juice from her tray. She was placed in the continuous tub every morning and spent the time while in this contrivance, singing silly ditties, inventing new words, and laughing uproariously at her own remarks. In seven weeks she was well, but failed to recall any of her experiences of the first three weeks at the hospital.

Symptoms of the Depressive Phase.—The symptoms of the depressive type of the affective disorders are exactly the opposite to those of mania. The patient now (1) has great difficulty in thinking, (2) is morbid in mood, and (3) shows psychomotor retardation. There are a labored effort to answer, a loss of ability to concentrate, and an inability to choose a direct line of action. The patient is tormented by a sense of insecurity, is overcome by a sense of guilt, and finds himself the prey of ideas of remorse and self-abasement. He complains of a total lack of affection; there is no relish for the things which formerly stirred him; he experiences the feeling that he is lost or being punished. There are an overpowering sense of futility, a "feeling of emptiness" and a desire to retreat from everything, to seek oblivion, and to end his life. Danger of suicide is the outstanding feature of this condition, and this alone justifies the greatest caution and consideration from the standpoint of care and treatment.

Types of Depression.—As in mania, there are different degrees of depression which are termed, respectively, (1) simple depression, (2) acute depression, and (3) stupor.

Simple Depression

The main features of this condition are those of mental and physical retardation. The patient has a haggard facial expression, conveying the impression of hopelessness. He speaks in a monotonous whisper and answers questions with but a few words. He shows no interest in anything about him, and sits with head bowed avoiding contact with others. He rarely admits being depressed but rather emphasizes a vague headache or insists that he is being punished for having committed various errors or misdemeanors in the past. He may also complain of insomnia, particularly in the early morning hours, or of loss of appetite and has a disposition to stay in bed or sit about overwhelmed by inertia and a sense of futility.

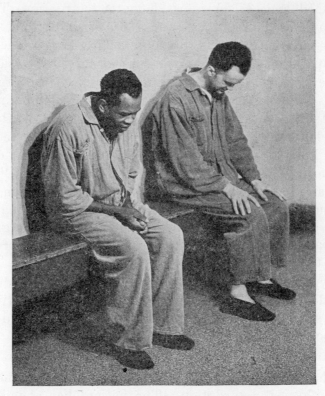

Fig. 7.—Two patients with mental depression showing the marked apathy and the characteristic posture.

Mrs. C. B., aged 29 years, married three years, had one child twenty-nine months old. Family history revealed nothing significant except that her father was a stolid, slow-going German who had a reputation for being a pessimist but was otherwise a stable, sober individual.

The patient had had a period of nervousness and depression. which lasted about three months, five years before. This was precipitated very suddenly by an unfortunate love affair. She

was then attending a summer course in education at a local
university where she met the young man in question. He had
encouraged her to believe he was greatly interested, but at the
school outing which terminated the summer session, he ignored
her and danced with another girl. The patient came home,
said little or nothing to her parents, and was found in bed
the following morning in a stupor. She had taken twelve
one-grain phenobarbital tablets. She was rushed to a hospital,
given emergency treatment, and then transferred to a nursing
home where she remained eight weeks.

The present attack began about six weeks before admission
to the psychopathic hospital. Again the onset was rather
abrupt. Her husband returned home from work one evening
and found her sobbing. After much urging on his part, she
confessed that she was crying because she was a bad mother
and a poor housekeeper. The husband naturally assured her
that she was quite the contrary but this only brought more
sobbing and self-depreciation. She worried excessively about
a small scar on the baby's temple which was caused by chicken
pox. She accused herself of "marking" the child. The family suspected that she was merely tired from her spring
housecleaning and hired a girl to come in and care for the
baby; her sister-in-law was called in to act as a companion.
For three weeks she remained at home, complaining of inability to concentrate, and she prayed a great deal of the
time. The well-meaning sister exhorted her frequently to
"snap out of it," and this merely served to agitate her. She
was finally taken to her parents in the country. On two occasions she was found walking along the country road, and
when questioned as to her destination she merely stated that
she wanted to "run away from everything." Her husband
came to visit her one Sunday afternoon and took her for an
auto ride back into the city. She requested him to stop at
the home, for she wanted some extra clothes for the baby.
She went to the kitchen, and, before the husband could
realize what she was about to do, she cut both her wrists
with a carving knife. She was brought directly to the psychopathic ward after emergency treatment of her wounds in the
accident room.

On the day of admission she was able to give a clear account of her actions but responded in a dull, apathetic manner.
She frequently interjected the remark that she should be
dead, but "I am too big a coward to take my own life." She
accused herself of being a rank failure and asserted that she

should never have been born. She cried but did not display many tears. She complained of a "numb" feeling in the head, of inability to sleep, and of a loss of appetite. The physical examination was entirely negative.

For three weeks she remained dull, indifferent, and spent a great deal of her time sitting in a dark corner of the hospital corridor, with her head bowed. She ate only when coaxed by the nurses. To every nurse she announced that there was no sense in bothering about her for she would die on the morrow. She never inquired about the welfare of her child and was rather indifferent about her husband's appearance during visiting hours. While she was not particularly untidy, she was rather slipshod in appearance and made no attempt to comb her hair or keep herself presentable. She became badly constipated and required daily enemas. She took little or no interest in ward activities and in her fellow patients.

In the fourth week of her hospital stay, she was given the first metrazol treatment. This was followed by four more, at the end of which she rapidly improved. Within two weeks she was clamoring for discharge, insisting that she must go home to take care of her family. She was cheerful and industrious, and in occupational therapy she was particularly adept in teaching English to a small group of foreign women.

Acute Depression

In acute depression as in acute mania, the symptoms develop with great suddenness. The impulsion to commit suicide is prominent; self-accusation and self-abasement are quickly demonstrated. There is an overpowering sense of utter futility. There is a delusional interpretation of physical disturbances and many queer ideas as to bodily functions are expressed. There are delusions of sin, the patient frequently accusing himself of being responsible for plagues, financial failures, and bad weather. These delusions are, however, in keeping with the morbid mood. The patient believes and insists on stating that he has been an impostor, that he is a man apart from everybody else, that he is only a living shell, etc. There may be fleeting hallucinations. There is always the conviction that the future is hopeless and that remedies are of no avail. The patient generally predicts for himself a horrible end and refuses food for the reason that he has no stomach or that his bodily organs are slowly petrifying. He has an anxious, hollow-eyed expression, and the skin becomes pale or sallow. Examination rarely reveals any serious physical disorder, although the patient generally loses considerable weight. Above all the impulsion to suicide is outstanding, and the patient may show a remarkable cunning in evading attendants and in carrying out his determination to end his sufferings.

Depressive Stupor

This represents the most severe degree of retardation and depression. The patient lies in bed, utterly indifferent to everything about him. He is mute, rarely showing any evidence that he understands what is being said and is entirely preoccupied with morbid and depressive ideas. He refuses all food and liquids. He may become incontinent, may develop bed sores, and always shows a progressive loss of weight. The patient is invariably constipated, has a foul breath and a coated tongue, and frequently develops an ascending infection of the urinary tract. The lips and finger tips may show a slight cyanosis; the pulse may be slow and soft; and on standing there may be a slight edema of the lower extremities. Such patients are so dull and stupid that they require bed care. Suicide is not a great potentiality because of the profound stupor and apathy, although vigilance should never be relaxed against this possibility.

H. C., a druggist 48 years old, was admitted because he refused to eat, lost interest in his work, and believed that he was dying of some horrible disease. He attempted suicide by taking poison.

He had been a sober, steady person of even temper, very industrious but inclined to worry more than he should. His mother had been confined to a state institution with melancholia at the time of her menopause. He himself had never been acutely ill before. Prior to his marriage he had had an operation for inguinal hernia. For twenty years he had managed a drug store which he owned and had developed a reputation for honesty, good nature, and exceptional skill in compounding prescriptions.

He prospered, and some eighteen months before his admission he ventured into the purchase of another drug store. This he did after much deliberation, for he was not inclined

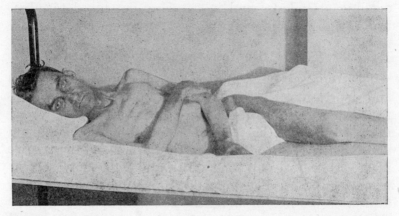

Fig. 8.—A stupor type of depression. Note the extreme emaciation due to self-starvation.

to take risks of any kind. Almost as soon as the transaction was completed, he became nervous and began to regret the step he had made. He became sleepless, talked incessantly of his poor judgment, and spent long hours over the books of the establishment. He expressed the opinion that he would lose everything and began to denounce himself for his recklessness. He lost weight and appetite and shortly became convinced that he had cancer of the stomach. Repeated examinations by many physicians and frequent assurances to the contrary failed to shake him of this belief. The day before his admission to the hospital, he disappeared behind his prescription counter and took a potion which consisted of a large amount of morphine and sodium amytal. He informed his assistant that he had taken poison. After being given emergency treatment in a neighborhood hospital, he was admitted to the psychopathic ward.

He was put to bed because he was emaciated, pale, and had a weak, slow pulse. However, he did not show many other signs of morphine poisoning. He was badly emaciated, the breath was foul, and the abdomen contained several hard masses which disappeared after a high enema. The bladder became distended, and catheterization was necessary for several weeks after admission.

He lay in a dull, depressed state with a sallow face and sunken, downcast eyes. He rarely answered any questions. Occasionally he responded after a long interval with a single, mumbled word. He absolutely ignored food, and tube feedings were necessary for many months. A superficial bed sore developed over the sacrum during the fifth week. The only movements he made were to rub his right hand over the right side of the head and to pull at the hair over this region. Eventually this portion of his scalp became practically bald of hair.

Not until the fourth month did he consent to eat, and then only when his wife fed him with his favorite dish which she prepared at home. He gradually took on weight, and it was then possible to communicate with him. He realized that he was in a hospital and insisted that he be sent to the county jail, for he believed himself to be a criminal. "It's utterly hopeless," was a frequent retort, "I have my right mind, but I can't think except with great effort. It takes me a long time to put my thoughts together. I know I've made a failure of my life, and I deserve all this punishment. I know I brought a great deal of misery to my wife and children."

For many months he continued to be mute, depressed, and self-accusatory. He maintained that he could not eat well because he had a "terrible blood disease" and that his stomach had decayed. He never showed any evidence of being hallucinated, and at all times was well oriented as to time and place. In the fourteenth month of his illness, after a rather discouraging prognosis was offered, he suddenly began to improve and within a few weeks was well enough to be discharged.

Circular Types

Some patients who suffer with a manic reaction may rapidly pass into a depressed state with but a few days or weeks of normal behavior in the intervening period. This circular form of mental disease may endure for years and hence, with the exception of short intervals of freedom, may require hospital care as a more or less chronic mental disease. For months on end the patient is in an exalted, talkative, and combative state, only to fall into a morbidly depressed, agitated mood during which he is suicidal and spends a great deal of time in retrospection and remorse over his unreasonable behavior during the manic phase.

Prognosis in Manic-Depressive Psychosis.—For a single episode of mania or depression the outlook is usually good, but recurrences are to be expected. However, second and third attacks need not necessarily occur in every case. An attack of mania in early adult life generally means many more attacks later. Depressions are more likely to occur in the later years of life.

It is never safe to predict the probable duration of any given attack, for there are great variations and even the same individual may have both short and long periods of mania and depression. The average for all manic attacks is about six months; for depressive episodes it is generally longer. When depressive periods show a strong element of fear, anxiety, and hypochondriasis, the disease may endure for many years. Likewise a mania may become chronic particularly in older individuals where it is associated with organic changes in the brain such as arteriosclerosis.

An outstanding feature of manic-depressive psychosis is the fact that even after repeated attacks the intellectual capacities are rarely impaired. In the free intervals the patient is usually able to carry on his regular occupation and live an entirely normal life.

Nursing Care of the Manic Phase.—It is doubtful whether even the mildest forms of hypomania can be adequately treated outside a mental institution. The exuberant energy of the exalted patient can rarely be dissipated without upsetting the relatives or irritating everyone with whom the patient comes in contact. The hypomanic is more a nuisance than he is a menace; he requires institutionalization not particularly for his own good, but for the good of society.

No greater degree of diplomacy and tact on the part of the nurse is called forth than that required to keep the hypomanic patient within bounds. He must be cajoled into obedience, and a little artful flattery may go a long way. The nurse must never commit herself to the patient to the effect that he is "normal," neither must she convey the impression that he is frankly insane. Firmness is always necessary, but this must be dispensed with an agreeable disposition and with the impression of tolerance and sympathy. Arguments should be avoided. An excellent way to placate the hypomanic patient is to allow him to write—of which he rarely tires—particularly encouraging the recording of memoirs or the writing of an autobiography.

In the more excited states of acute mania where the pressure of activity is great, the situation calls for various sedative measures. Prolonged baths, in specially designed tubs and of slightly lower than body temperature, are favorite procedures in many modern institutions. If the patient is greatly disturbed, the immersion may be for eight hours daily. Wet packs are even more effective in inducing relaxation, although there may be difficulty in getting the patient to cooperate, and occasionally the excitement incidental to the treatment may not justify this procedure. Hydrotherapy may be supplemented by hypnotics which, however, should be administered in small doses at regular intervals. Paraldehyde in doses of 2 to 4 drams, 30 grains of chloral hydrate, or 1½ grains of phenobarbital are recommended as being most desirable.

Special Treatment of the Manic Phase.—A treatment of mania which has met with favor during the past eight years is that which is known as the *deep narcosis therapy.* In this country sodium amytal is usually selected for this purpose. The patient should be in good physical condition before this procedure is attempted. Three grains of sodium amytal are given by mouth every three or four hours during the first day, and this is increased daily for about four days, so that the patient is maintained in a somnolent state during that period for fifteen or twenty hours a day. After a deep sleep has been assured a fixed dosage is given by mouth or rectum for six more days. After the tenth day each daily dose is reduced by one-half, and all medications cease on the fourteenth day. The patient should be allowed to sleep preferably on a comfortable mattress laid on the floor so that restraint is avoided and the danger of falling out of bed is obviated. In the event that the patient develops signs of cyanosis, the treatment should be abruptly discontinued. The pulse, respirations, and blood pressure should be carefully observed. In case of circulatory collapse or slow, shallow, irregular respiration, strychnine is kept at hand for immediate hypodermic use. During the semistupor induced by the continued narcosis, the patient is in a state of toxic confusion and may give expression to ideas which throw considerable light on some of the contributing and unconscious factors leading to the manic excitement. These should be carefully recorded by the nurse, for they may have considerable psychotherapeutic value in the later adjustment of the patient to his personal problems.

In recent years, several clinics have tried the metrazol convulsion treatment in abating the manic excitement. In a large percentage of manic patients a series of several metrazol convulsions may lead to such a complete remission of the manic symptoms that relatives often believe the patient is cured. However, this freedom from excitement is usually short-lived, never being longer than ten days, and such treatment does not shorten the length of the entire manic cycle. Because of the serious complications which often follow the metrazol convulsion, this radical treatment is not advocated in any but the most violent forms.

Nursing Care of the Depressive Phase.—As in mania, so in depression, hospitalization is the wisest procedure. Possibly the mild or simple forms of depression in selected cases may be adequately treated at home. As a rule, relatives of patients with depression make willing but inefficient nurses. They are prone to exhort the depressed individual to "snap out of it" because they entertain the belief that he is simply tired and merely needs a change of scenery. Moreover, because the patient's mind is "clear," a mental hospital is believed to be detrimental. Not until the patient steadily resists feeding or makes an attempt at suicide is the real gravity of the situation thoroughly appreciated.

The basic principle in the nursing care of any melancholia is to reduce life to a very simple level. In the early stages of the disease, the patient should be asked to do nothing which requires concerted thinking or demands critical decisions. Where nourishment is refused, tube feeding is in order, but this need not be done more than twice a day or even once daily. It is absolutely necessary to keep the bowels carefully regulated. Intestinal stasis is very frequently associated with the general physical and mental apathy. Every caution should be taken to avoid infection and any abrasion or ulceration of the skin should be protected by antisepsis and sterile dressings. Foci of infection, such as bad teeth, have been considered as factors, but there is no good evidence that extraction of infected teeth has a beneficial effect upon the depressed state.

No matter how mild a depression may appear, and no matter how disarming the patient's assurance that he will do himself no harm, the danger of suicide is outstanding. Unremitting supervision both day and night is absolutely necessary. A depressed patient should not be left alone for any reason whatsoever. The nurse should be on guard against every strategy which such a patient may utilize to carry out his purpose. Suicidal impulsions are likely to develop suddenly and may pass in the same abrupt fashion. Hanging by a bedsheet, cutting the wrists with a small fragment of glass, setting fire to the clothing with a concealed match, and jumping into an unguarded tub of scalding hot water are some of the techniques of self-destruction which are engineered by the suicidal patient. The supervision of the depressed individual should be adequate, but at the same time, it should be exercised in a casual and tactful manner, so that it does not become a form of intolerable scrutiny.

Sleeplessness in depressed patients is a common and difficult problem. Because of the apathy and inactivity, a normal amount of sleep is probably not absolutely necessary. Many of these patients complain of shallow sleep and of insomnia, particularly in the very early hours of the morning. Hence, a sedative with a prolonged or delayed action is recommended, such as veronal, 10 to 15 grains, or phenobarbital in doses of 1 to 3 grains at bedtime.

When the depressed condition improves sufficiently to allow some degree of cooperation, occupational therapy is of unquestioned benefit. Not only does it tend to arouse normal interests, but it engenders a feeling of creative success and aids in reestablishing the self-confidence and self-esteem which are so sadly lacking in the melancholic individual.

Equally important is the necessity of giving the patient a better understanding of his temperament and personality. An open discussion of the patient's personal affairs, particularly emphasizing the situations which have acted as immediate factors in causing his illness, is as important as the purely physical phases of the treatment.

Medical and Special Treatment of Depression.—Many drugs have been administered with the hope of elevating the depressed individual out of his dejection, but few have proved to have any consistent value. Of these perhaps benzedrine or amphetamine sulphate has been most popular and, in some cases of mild depression, has been beneficial. A 10 mg. tablet is usually given in the morning and another at noon.

Far more successful and in many cases decidedly miraculous in its effects has been convulsion-producing shock therapy either with metrazol or the electric current. A series of six to eight convulsions will frequently relieve the worst symptoms of depression and will induce the patient to assume a radically different and even optimistic attitude—a complete reversal of personality. Morbid ideas are no longer expressed, animation reappears and sleep and appetite become normal.

The technique of these treatments is described in another chapter. Because electric shock is less harmful and more easily administered, it has displaced the metrazol treatment in most hospitals of this country. This therapy has been reported as being successful in over 80 per cent of cases treated.

References

Association for Research in Nervous and Mental Disease: Manic De-
    pressive Psychosis, Baltimore, 1931, Williams & Wilkins Co.
Brown, Henry C.: A Mind Mislaid, New York, 1937, E. P. Dutton &
    Co.
Jayson, Lawrence M.: Mania, New York, 1937, Funk & Wagnalls Co.
Muncie, Wendell: Psychobiology and Psychiatry, St. Louis, 1939, The C.
    V. Mosby Company.

Questions for Chapter VIII

Affective Reaction Types—The Manic Depressive Psychoses

1. Describe the syntonic temperament.
2. What is the meaning of the term ''affective reaction''?
3. Explain the difference between constitutional and reactive depressions.
4. What are the three outstanding symptoms of the manic phase?
5. Describe ''elated mood.''
6. Differentiate briefly between three types of mania.
7. Discuss the symptomatology of a manic patient as to orientation, powers of judgment and reasoning, presence of hallucinations and delusions, physical and mental activity.
8. What are three degrees of depression?
9. Why must depressed patients be watched constantly?
10. What is meant by the circular type of manic-depressive psychosis?
11. What qualifications of personality are necessary in a nurse caring for manic patients?
12. Would it be easy to distract the manic patient's attention from undesirable to desirable activity? Describe a few methods of doing so.
13. Give a brief summary of the nursing care of a depressed patient.
14. For what phase would continuous tub therapy be used? Deep narcosis? Metrazol therapy? Electric shock? Discuss these treatments.

CHAPTER IX

AFFECTIVE REACTION TYPES— INVOLUTIONAL PSYCHOSES

The involutional period, which begins roughly about the forty-second year in women and about ten years later in men, is accompanied by extensive but gradual changes in practically all the organs of the body. Some of these changes are only vaguely understood, but it appears certain that the reproductive organs suffer a decrease in activity which is particularly evident in women. Here the involutional period is announced by the cessation of menstruation and by certain nervous and vegetative disturbances which are grouped together under the term *menopause syndrome*. This syndrome occurs in many women, and ordinarily is of no great significance, its effect passing away within a few months or a year to leave little or no permanent nervous disorder. The symptoms consist of the well-known "hot flashes," excessive sweating, headache, nervous irritability, and some degree of insomnia. It is fairly well established that such a condition is due largely to the sudden lack of ovarian hormone, estrin, in the blood, and injections of this principle promptly relieve these symptoms.

Causes.—The true involutional psychoses are based on deeper and more complicated factors than a mere diminution of sexual and endocrine activity, although one must concede that these play a minor or aggravating role. Probably more important are various temperamental and psychological elements in the personality of those who suffer with mental upset at the involutional period. A review of the life history of most of these patients reveals certain traits, habits, and dispositions

117

which merely become exaggerated to the point where they must be regarded as abnormal. People who have lived narrow social lives, who have been overmeticulous, sensitive, rigid in their daily habits, colorless and frugal; women who have been known to be excessively jealous, suspicious, and sexually frigid are particularly prone to some mental distortion in the involutional years. Excessive worriers, fussy, apprehensive individ-

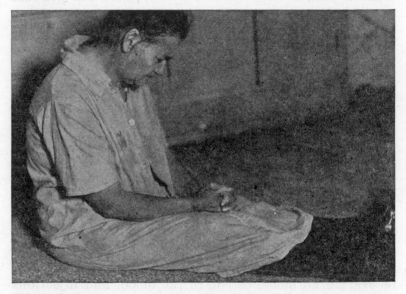

Fig. 9.—Involutional melancholia. The patient seeks the darkest corridor of the ward and sits in dejected fashion upon the floor.

uals, and those with compulsive behavior may show increased agitation, anxiety, and depression during this critical period. In short, any situation characterized by a chronic sense of ego insecurity is a definite factor.

To these underlying causes are added the immediate strains and problems which act as exciting causes. The death of a relative on whom the patient was particularly dependent, behavior of misguided sons and daughters, financial troubles, and the breaking up of the home are commonly found to be the immediate psychic causes.

Symptoms.—Every psychotic symptom may appear, but an undercurrent depression or anxiety with a tendency to general uneasiness and self-depreciation seems to be present in most cases. It is the depression feature which has led to the term "involutional melancholia." For a time it was believed that the disease was merely another variety of manic-depressive psychosis, and, for that matter in a few cases, the depressed phase which appears in the involutional period may be merely a duplication of previous attacks of manic-depressive psychosis. However, in most instances the agitation, the delusions of sin, the extreme hypochondriasis appearing for the first time at the involutional period constitute a definite and separate clinical picture.

The disease generally develops in an insidious fashion. The patient becomes peevish, sleepless, has unprovoked spells of weeping, complains of a feeling of pressure in the head, and worries excessively about minor matters. Obsessive preoccupation with some trifling misdemeanor committed some time in the past, a desire to confess unpardonable sins, and a marked agitation with weeping and wringing of the hands announce the acute phase of the mental upset. The patient feels that there is no hope, that she will be jailed and put to death. Suicidal impulsions are frequently demonstrated in spite of the appeals for help. The patient refuses to eat because she has no stomach or intestines, or because the food is poisoned. So-called nihilistic delusions which deny the existence of things which no longer interest the patient, such as home, husband, and children, are outstanding. With all this agitation, the patient usually realizes that he or she is ill; orientation is good and memory is not badly impaired.

Classification of Involution Psychoses.—The depressed and agitated types, unquestionably the most common forms, are called **involutional melancholia.** A smaller number of patients develop no great degree of depression, show little anxiety, but react with delusions of reference and persecution whereby they project their sense of insecurity on external situations. This form of involutional psychosis is called the **paranoid type** and develops in men and women who have been notably self-centered, suspicious, jealous, and unforgiving types. The outlook in this form is rather poor.

A brief résumé of patients demonstrating these two types of mental disease will illustrate the important features in each. The first patient described is typical of the **melancholic form.**

M. S., a Slavish housewife forty-seven years old, was admitted in a badly agitated condition, wringing her hands, crying, and demanding that the priest be called so that she might confess her many sins. The right forearm and hand were covered with frayed bandages at which the patient was continually picking.

The patient was born in Austria and came to this country with her husband twenty-six years ago. She was the mother of five children, had always lived in a foreign neighborhood, had few outside interests except those centering about the Catholic church which she attended every Sunday. For twenty years she had not missed a single early mass. She was a meticulous housewife, rather fussy and fretful with her children who regarded her as strict and old-fashioned. She learned little or no English, had nothing to do with the neighbors except to give them a nod of recognition, but kept a colorful flower garden. She wore clothing which was consistently outmoded and refused to allow her growing children to don any modern or fashionable dress. She particularly tyrannized her oldest daughter whom she regarded as being somewhat incorrigible. Five years prior to her present illness her husband lost his job in the steel mills, and she eked out the family income by doing day work four days a week. During this interval she scarcely spoke to her husband or to the older children and insisted on managing all the family finances to the last penny, because she was now the "wage earner."

Six months before her admission the oldest daughter obtained a position as a housemaid but came home abruptly because of pernicious vomiting which proved to be due to pregnancy. The patient at once became badly agitated, discon-

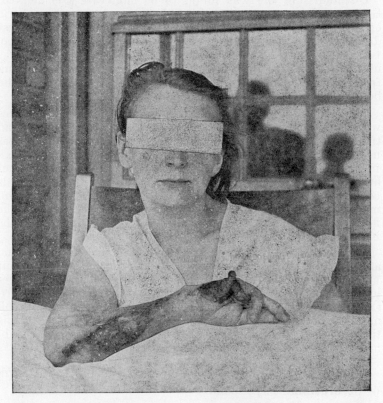

Fig. 10.—Self-mutilation in involutional melancholia. The entire forearm along the ulnar surface was picked away and the little finger was practically amputated.

tinued her work, and sat in the back yard all day wringing her hands, and picking at her right forearm. She called for the priest, who came but failed to console her. She visited the church several times a day, and finally the priest referred her to a physician. She refused to go, instead cried out that she had committed horrible sins and that the church had disowned her. A neighbor recommended a Christian Science practitioner whom she consulted every day for several weeks. During the course of the "treatment" the patient continued to tear at the forearm until the area was eroded as far up as the elbow.

On admission she was found to be moderately emaciated. Because of language difficulties she was able to give little or no information. She stated that her husband and oldest daughter were dead and that shortly she would be dead, too, because she was a "bad woman." The right forearm was ulcerated down to the muscle tissues over an area extending from the elbow to the little finger which was eroded to the bone on the distal phalanx.

She refused to eat and was badly constipated; her eyes were dark and deep sunken. She insisted that the bowels had turned to stone and that her heart was also petrified. It was necessary to restrain her in order to maintain adequate dressings on the right arm. She attempted suicide by banging her head against the marble partitions in the washroom. Periods of extreme agitation alternated with periods of stupor and mutism during which she sat in the darkest corridor on the floor with head bowed; occasionally she barked to convey the impression that she was a dog.

Six months after admission she no longer picked at the arm, ate sparingly, but still insisted that she would be soon "put under the ground." She willingly ate fruit if it was fed to her by her 11-year-old daughter. Three months later she admitted the identity of her husband, became cooperative, and took natural interest in her work in the ward kitchen. At this time a sister died, she attended the funeral, showed no abnormal reactions, and was shortly discharged as recovered.

The following history is typical of the paranoid form of **involutional psychosis**:

H. S., a schoolteacher aged 43 years, was admitted because she accused the neighbors of poisoning her with noxious gases and because she believed her husband was intimate with a 15-year-old girl in the neighborhood.

Of Scotch extraction, she was born on a farm in southern Ohio, was reared in a strict Presbyterian household, was greatly attached to her father, and was somewhat jealous of her brother who was a few years older, a better scholar and more popular with his schoolmates. Very early in adolescence she showed signs of sensitivity and frequently reported that her friends were talking about her. Her first teaching assignment was in a small country school. She was discharged because she was too harsh with the older pupils but came home with the story that she resigned because the chairman of the board tried to make advances to her. Two years later she obtained a position in a larger, consolidated school in a nearby town, where she lived with a widower uncle. She maintained her position for eighteen years. By her fellow-teachers she was regarded as a touchy, suspicious woman whom they tactfully avoided when they could. When she was 35 years old, she married a farmer ten years her senior. Shortly thereafter the uterus was removed because of fibroid tumors. She returned to work after several months of convalescence and shortly complained to the principal that her substitute was an indiscreet woman because she had left some "love notes" and a lipstick in the desk.

When she was admitted, she appeared somewhat haughty and indignant but refused to answer any questions referring to her personal affairs. She appeared well oriented and her memory for general events was good. She insisted that she was well and advised the ward physician to look into her neighbors and her husband if he desired information. From the husband it was learned that she had been delusional for several years; she had never displayed any normal sex desire, was very jealous of his sister, and upbraided him whenever he conversed casually with anyone of the opposite sex. For the past six months she had been accusing him of "carrying on" with a 15-year-old girl who clerked in a confectionery store at the neighboring corner, where he was accustomed to buy tobacco. She claimed she sensed the odor of the young girl's perfumery on his person. Lately she had detected other strange odors in the house and concluded that the neighbors had been "valving poison gas" through her basement windows. She neglected her housework, refused to touch her husband's linen, and washed only her own. She had been reading several books on "spiritualism."

On the wards she was cleanly, fairly cooperative, but definitely tight-lipped and seclusive. Several times she complained to the head nurse that the food tasted bad, and she refused her meals for several days at a time. She accused a pupil nurse of "making eyes" at her husband when he was being escorted from the ward. She frequently demanded her release, but rarely pressed the matter with any argument.

Her condition remained unimproved for many months, and she was finally committed to a state hospital.

Prognosis.—The outlook for the agitated and depressed types of involutional psychosis is fairly good,

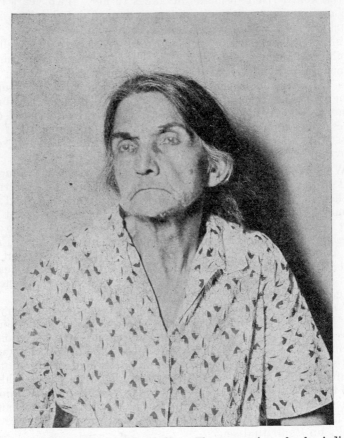

Fig. 11.—Involutional melancholia. The expression clearly indicates the internal miseries of the patient, being those of sorrow, anxiety and despair.

particularly if the prepsychotic personality is not badly warped. Approximately 80 per cent of such patients improve, although recovery may not take place until after as many as eight years. In the paranoid form the prospects of recovery are practically nil, and the patient suffers a gradual but progressive deterioration, not unlike that of schizophrenia, which the condition greatly resembles.

Nursing Care of Involutional Melancholia.—The average case of involutional melancholia is best treated in

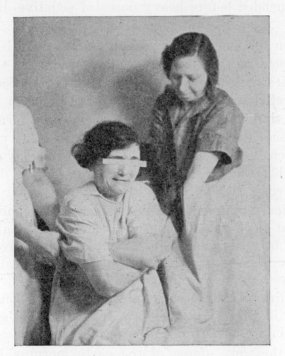

Fig. 12.—Agitated state in involutional melancholia.

a mental institution although milder forms can be handled at home under the care of experienced nurses. Every precaution and procedure which has been emphasized in the management of a depressed phase of manic-depressive psychosis applies in these cases as well. The greatest danger is always the possibility of suicide. Tube feeding is necessary in a large proportion of these cases in the more acute phase of the illness, after which the patient will generally eat without coertion. Complete rest in bed is recommended and the patient should be spared from any activity requiring initiative, concentrative effort or physical overexertion. In states of extreme agitation, a continuous tub bath is recommended before heavy doses of sedative drugs are given.

When the melancholic patient shows a consistent improvement in appetite, shows more interest in the ward activities and is less morose and agitated, recovery is accelerated and the management of the patient becomes vastly simpler by the application of some form of occupational therapy. Sewing, weaving or any constructive theme which calls for a continuous display of interest rather than a sudden burst of energy is definitely indicated.

Medical Treatment of Involutional Melancholia.—The barbital and bromide sedatives should not be given too freely because these are highly accumulative. Frequently when allowed to take her own medication, the woman with involutional melancholia will develop a semidelirious state because of drug intoxication. Probably it is safer to give chloral hydrate, in 10 gr. doses three times a day if agitation is too great.

For the wakefulness of the early morning hours, a delayed action principle such as "an enseal" or coated seconal tablet is particularly useful.

There has been much discussion in reference to the value of the ovarian hormone in the treatment of involutional melancholia. If the patient suffers with "hot flashes" and other subjective symptoms typical of the menopause, the administration by injection of 2,000 to

10,000 international units of estrin in oil has specific value. Whether or not estrin has any positive effect on the deeper mental disorders of the involutional period is still an open question. It is unwise to give estrin to older women who have passed the menopause by five or ten years. The same arguments apply in reference to the use of stilbestrol.

Decidedly more beneficial in treating the apathy and depression of involutional melancholia is shock therapy with metrazol or with the electric current. Some writers report that as high as 80 per cent of the patients recover or show marked improvement with this form of treatment. Generally a favorable response occurs after the fifth or sixth convulsion. If no improvement occurs after the tenth treatment, shock therapy should be discontinued for a period of several weeks and a second series administered. The contraindications and complications attending shock therapy are discussed in a separate chapter.

Psychosurgery as a Treatment of Melancholia.—In severe, chronic forms of agitated melancholia, where shock treatment has little or no value, a rather radical procedure called pre-frontal lobotomy was introduced in 1935 by two Portuguese clinicians, Moniz and Lima. In this country, the technique has been refined and carefully studied by Drs. Freeman and Watts of Washington. The procedure consists of bluntly cutting through the nerve tracts passing from the frontal lobes to the thalamus or feeling tone centers.

The results appear to be decidedly beneficial; the patient not only becomes free of the emotionally painful element in his self-preoccupation, but actually takes on a happy and carefree attitude. Personality changes thus produced make the patient somewhat less responsible, but in many instances, a routine occupation can be successfully resumed. Where the results are not as startling, the patient is at least less difficult to manage and is rendered more cooperative.

References

Freeman, Walter, and Watts, James W.: Psychosurgery, Springfield, Ill., 1942, Charles C. Thomas.

Mayer and Goldstein: Clinical Endocrinology of the Female, Philadelphia, 1932, W. B. Saunders Co.

Noyes, Arthur: Modern Clinical Psychiatry, ed. 2, Philadelphia, 1939, W. B. Saunders Co.

Rety, Joseph: Transition Years, New York, 1940, Greenberg, Publisher, Inc.

Questions for Chapter IX

Affective-Reaction Types—Involutional Psychoses

1. What is the "involutional period"?
2. What are the symptoms of the menopause syndrome?
3. Discuss the causes and symptoms of the involutional psychoses.
4. Describe a typical case of involutional melancholia.
5. What are nihilistic delusions?
6. What is the significant symptom in the paranoid type of involutional psychosis?
7. How can the agitation of the involutional psychosis be controlled?
8. What danger is present in melancholic states?
9. What value has estrin in the treatment of involutional melancholia?
10. Discuss the prognosis in involutional psychosis.
11. What type of treatment is most specific and valuable in cases of involutional melancholia?
12. Describe briefly what is done in psychosurgery to the brain matter. When should one advise such a radical procedure?

Curare - Used by Indians on arrowheads -

Helps relax muscles in surgical work -

Acts on motor end plate -

Symptoms - Haziness of eyes - Facial muscles start showing -

I. V. acts in 2 min.

I.M. " " 20 "

1cc of curare = 20 mgm. Give 1 mgm for 2 pounds of weight -

Antidote - Prostigmine - 1-20,000

CHAPTER X

SCHIZOPHRENIC REACTION TYPES

In the normal person feelings which arise to consciousness have a certain appropriateness and predictability. It is natural to feel gay on a festive occasion and to show sadness as a response to a death or tragedy. It is natural to display anger at times, to feel dismay, surprise, fear, to rise in sympathy to a feeling of indignation, to show love and compassion. Such affect is characteristic of the average individual and, as we have seen, is exaggerated in the syntonic person who is prone to manic-depressive psychosis.

There are individuals in whom this capacity to feel with others is lacking or is weakened. These people have a poverty of affect, or, when they display it, they do it in an awkward, inappropriate manner. In this sense, they are unpredictable, seem often to be without passion or feeling, are rather dry and indifferent, and may show a mood which is not ordinarily in keeping with the thoughts of the moment. Such people are prone to withdraw from normal human contacts and definitely seem to lack the proper herd instinct. They are frequently termed *schizoids*. They are unusually shy and sensitive, lack a sense of humor, and are inclined to be suspicious, cold, and always a little eccentric.

This lack of natural human warmth may appear in the young person entering adolescence. It announces itself by an overseriousness, painful self-consciousness and a tendency to prefer one's own company. The individual becomes unduly preoccupied by daydreams and fantasies which are preferred to the problems of reality.

Mental capacity is generally normal, but there is an abnormal interest in dry philosophies, solitary pursuits, long walks, or in nature study. Toward the opposite sex there is little of the emotional attitude which is normal for young people. Instead there may be an eccentric display of interest in someone with whom there has been little or no natural contact. In the face of a minor or major tragedy involving some member of the family, there is often little or no show of normal affect while some trivial situation may bring out a wild surge of excitement. It is this type of individual who is prone to develop schizophrenia.

Definition.—Schizophrenia, or dementia precox, is a psychosis which appears as a garbled reaction on the part of an individual who lacks the deep instinctual capacities and feelings in meeting the acute problems of reality. There is either a total lack of normal affect or a perversion of the emotions and with this a tendency to withdraw into a world of one's own subjective construction. The disease may develop at any age, but the greatest number of its victims are found in the adolescent and earliest adult periods of life between the seventeenth and the twenty-fifth year.

Etiology.—The true etiology of this disease is unknown. For a time it was believed to have an organic basis, but no consistently uniform brain changes have been demonstrated. The victims of schizophrenia, it may be said, do generally have a thin body, are likely to be angular in build and of delicate bony architecture, a bodily type which Kretschmer calls the "asthenic" constitution. That heredity is an important factor is demonstrated in the finding that 50 per cent of the patients have a family record of mental breakdown. Probably the average psychiatrist of today believes that

30, 40 thousand people are affected by schizophrenia a year.

1/4 of all hosp. new admissions is schizophrenia

schizophrenia represents a type of serious personality disorganization, an abnormal response to environmental troubles by one in whom there is a lack of harmony between thought, feeling, and behavior.

Symptoms of Schizophrenia.—The disease may have a slow onset, frequently developing over a long period of months or years. Occasionally the major symptoms may break out in an abrupt fashion. Ordinarily there are progressive indifference to normal interests, blunting of the emotions, and a sullen, suspicious attitude. Odd and unpredictable behavior, silly postures, excessive preoccupation with trivial things are common symptoms. Attempts to bring the patient back to a normal concern and interest in what is going on about him may only produce silly laughter, a stolid indifference, or a sudden and unexpected outburst of violence.

There is soon manifested a disharmony between thought and feeling. While talking of something which ordinarily would be associated with sorrow, the patient may emit an empty laugh or may burst into tears when discussing some casual affair. There seems to be no ability to appreciate natural joy, sorrow, or fear.

Sooner or later the schizophrenic patient expresses ideas of persecution, and ordinary events are explained as having a particularly significant reference to him. His mind is being "read" by those about him, and passers-by are talking about him. He re-enforces his beliefs by stating that he hears voices (hallucinations) denouncing him or controlling his behavior. In response to these voices he may become impulsive and unpredictable in his behavior. Reality and unreality are no longer differentiated, and there may suddenly develop wild panic, confusion, marked antagonism and resistance to admonition or assurance. The patient may quickly retreat into a stoic silence and a frozen immobility and may stand for hours in a fixed attitude, mute, resistive, and with a stony expression on the face.

Just as suddenly the patient may become quiet, almost normal, and may then demonstrate that his mental faculties are good, memory is intact, and general intelligence is unimpaired. Judgment, however, is poor, and generally the patient is not particularly aware of his abnormal behavior or its effect on others about him. This mental disorder has many other features; in general it means a serious disintegration of personality, for the symptoms are grounded on a fundamental defect in the instinctual spheres. Social adaptation is extremely deficient, there is a turning away from reality, a complete domination of the individual by his twisted instincts and a tendency to a return to certain childish or infantile modes of thinking and behavior.

Types of Schizophrenia.—Kraepelin, the German psychiatrist, recognized four types of schizophrenia. This classification implies not so much a different mental picture in each type, but rather points out the different methods whereby the individual attempts to compensate for his feelings of instinctual inadequacy and his desire to maintain some degree of inner comfort and freedom from painful self-consciousness and unconscious conflict.

The four types are as follows: (1) schizophrenia simplex, (2) hebephrenia, (3) catatonia and (4) the paranoid form.

Simple Type

In this condition the patient manifests his defects by being simply a colorless and disinterested person. He lives in idle fantasy, content to lead a simple, shiftless life without ambition. Interests are small; there seems to be no great concern over important events and no great desire to assume any responsibility. Conversation is scant and trivial, and the individual prefers his own company and rarely shows any interest in the opposite

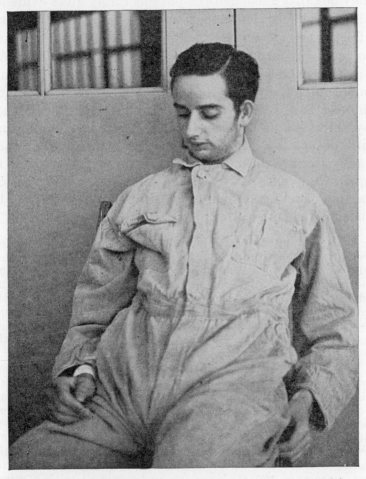

Fig. 13.—A young man with the simple type of schizophrenia. He lacks ambition and interest, is content to sit alone and has no great concern about his personal appearance.

sex. Normal heterosexual development and social instincts seem to be lacking. Occasionally there may be

periods of unrest and irritability, but these are short-
lived and the patient sinks more and more into a dull,
apathetic state. In spite of this torpor, the intellect
may be fairly good, and the patient rarely gives evidence
of delusions or hallucinations. Nonetheless, the total
effect is that of a queer person who is inaccessible, hard
to get acquainted with, and decidedly uninteresting. We
are all acquainted with such people. They manage some-
how to live their monotonous lives as menials, servants,
harvest hands, and vagrants who eke out an existence
by doing simple things or working at some simple routine occupation. If they have any special gifts, they
rarely display them, or they lack the aggressiveness to
apply them successfully. The following is a fairly good
sample of a simple type of schizophrenia as it may be
encountered in practice.

J. P., a boy 17 years old, tall, lanky, and a little under-
weight, was brought to the psychiatric clinic by his mother
who was greatly concerned over his lack of ambition and his
indisposition to finish his education. His parents are both
educated people, the mother being a schoolteacher and the
father an attorney. There were no decidedly abnormal traits
in either parent, except that the father is a tall, gaunt, quiet-
spoken man who rarely displays any great emotion even in the
courtroom.

The patient had always been a quiet, conscientious student
until his junior year in high school, when he began neglecting
his school work because he spent a great deal of time prac-
ticing with the high school band. He played the trombone
very well and was selected to participate in a national contest.
He joined no social clubs at school and outside his musical
activities chose to come home after school and listen to the
radio. He failed in two subjects in his third year, and after
two months in the senior class he became ill with a minor
throat ailment after which he refused to return to school. He
took to sleeping late, getting up in a languid manner, eating
sparingly, and spending long hours just sitting in a rocking
chair, smoking many cigarettes and staring into space. His
mother, sensing that something was wrong, left him to his own

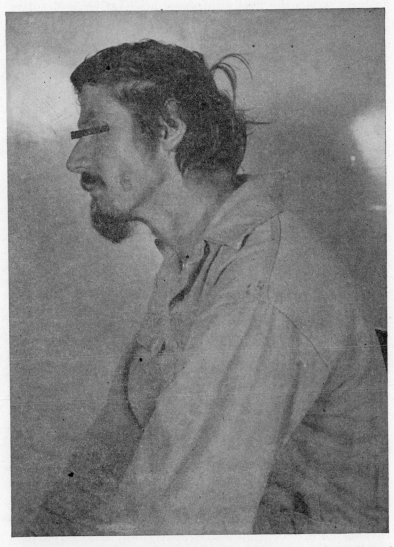

Fig. 14.—A patient who is schizophrenic and who, as an expression of his poor social adaptability, retreated into an ascetic, hermit-like existence, taking on the gaunt, bearded appearance of a religious zealot. He encouraged the belief that he was a great prophet.

devices. When she finally informed.him that he need not return to school, he felt vastly relieved. Gradually he gave up his trombone playing and became interested in fixing radio equipment at home. He spent the afternoons in long solitary walks or on his bicycle. After supper which he ate without comment, he left the house again to wander along about the streets until late hours. He never inquired about his parents' welfare, and to all the entreaties of his parents as to his lack of concern for his future he responded with stony silence and a stolid indifference. He had no ambitions and admitted that he did not care about his lack of education. When his mother burst into tears, he showed no evidence of emotion. He saw no occasion for the conference with the physician and apparently took no interest in what was going on. He co-operated rather indifferently during the examination and answered all questions in a monotonous voice and with short, colorless responses. There were no evidence of hallucinosis, no delusions, and no memory defects, but he showed no normal attention. Normal feelings were lacking, there was neither joy nor sorrow, no anxiety or irritability demonstrated during the entire procedure.

Hebephrenic Type

This form of schizophrenia occurs at an early age and represents a more severe disintegration of personality than do the other types. Patients who develop hebephrenia are young people who have been unmistakably queer and overscrupulous about trivial things, and who have been particularly given to brooding over religious and obscure philosophies while their normal schoolmates indulge in natural play and social activity.

Ideas of reference are commonly expressed; normal contact with others seems distasteful; and the patients give themselves over to phantasies and to long periods of seclusiveness. A silly smile or shallow laughter on little or no provocation is frequently noted as the earliest sign of true mental breakdown. Hallucinations of sight and hearing are invariably demonstrated. Peculiar mannerisms appear, which are repeated over and over again; speech becomes incoherent; and the patient becomes pro-

gressively indifferent to relatives and to the normal activities of the household. Outbursts of anger, obscene
behavior and a frank absence of any modesty or sense

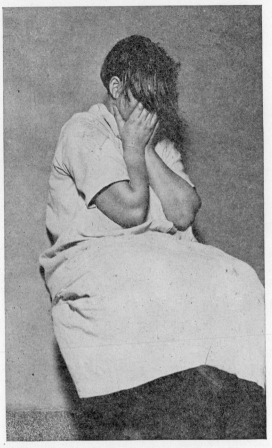

Fig. 15.—Schizophrenia of the hebephrenic type. This young woman
conceals her silly smile behind her unkempt hair and her hands. She is
seclusive, silly and negativistic.

of shame indicate that the patient no longer cares to
maintain self-esteem and is content to revert to silly,
childish levels of behavior and responsibility. This process of retreating into infantile levels of reaction and

into a life entirely dominated by phantasy is called *regression*. A case history will present more adequately the story of this type of personality disintegration.

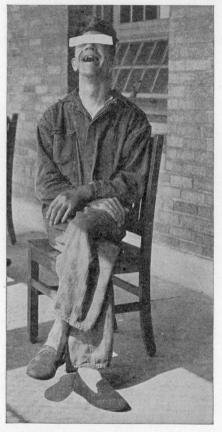

Fig. 16.—The silly behavior of hebephrenia. The patient laughs boisterously and without provocation.

F. B. was only 19 years old when she was admitted to the psychopathic hospital. The daughter of missionary parents, she was born in a West African Mission Station. The father was a quiet-spoken man, definitely esthetic and highly principled, having little patience with sensual matters and naturally very pious and religious. The girl's mother was better balanced in this respect, was more practical and tolerant, but entirely dominated by her husband.

The patient, herself, had an abnormal social development during the first seven years of her life, in that her only playmates were native African children. Toward them, naturally, she had always taken an attitude of superiority. On entering a boarding school in this country, she had great difficulty with her classmates who regarded her as a little "queer and superior." She was inclined to be a little too critical with them and insisted on dictating to them too much about personal matters. In her twelfth year she had a long siege of pneumonia after which she lost weight, was chronically anemic and undernourished. She spent long hours in prayer, wrote endless letters to her parents in Africa, most of them consisting of long quotations from the Bible. She insisted on wearing her oldest and shoddiest clothing to the schoolroom and bitterly criticized her classmates for not doing likewise.

Her social behavior improved somewhat in her high school years, but she made few friends. She had a dog to whom she was greatly attached and spent most of her free time in his company, taking long walks. She showed a preference for mathematics and biblical history. Menstruation did not begin until she was sixteen years old and then was very irregular. There was a moderate overgrowth of hair on the upper lip.

She entered the freshman year of college some eleven months before her admission to the hospital. While her scholastic record was good, she was known as being definitely a queer girl who avoided company, smiled a great deal to herself, and had no interest in the opposite sex. Her parents, while on furlough from Africa, visited her during the Christmas holidays, and her mother expressed fears that she was not in good mental health. She manifested no great enthusiasm over their appearance, in spite of the fact that she had not seen them for over five years. During the commencement festivities she disappeared from the campus for several days and later her guardian learned that she had spent the time at an evangelical camp meeting. She remained on the campus during the summer months to take some advanced courses in mathematics. During this interval she roomed with two other young women in the house of one of the faculty members. The latter were in the habit of discussing their love affairs in her presence, and in these discourses she suddenly manifested an unusual interest. Among other things, she inquired about various matters of sex and how to approach members of the opposite sex. A few nights later she informed one of the girls that she saw the face of her future husband in the stovepipe which she scrutinized for several hours during which she sat in a state of entrancement with a silly smile on her face. Early the next morning she accosted a 13-year-old newsboy and informed him that she would marry him that very day. When he made light of this proposal, she became infuriated, struck him in the face, and chased him off the premises. Returning to her room, she tore down the stovepipe, thereby burning her hands, tore off her clothing, and became utterly unmanageable.

On being admitted she refused to answer the questions asked by the nurse. Both hands were badly blistered. She tore open several vesicles before her hands were bandaged and she was restrained. She smiled in a silly manner and identified the house physician as "Herbert." She insisted on having the window opened because "they are playing the Wedding March." Her speech was utterly incoherent; she was definitely hallucinated, admitting hearing voices which questioned her moral purity.

During several days of restraint she continued to talk incoherently. Out of this incoherency one could make out that she was phantasizing a courtship in which she was the central character. She carried on an endless dialogue, at one time representing the lover, at another time the maiden who was ardently courted. After this she entered a long period of silence, during which she was mute, resistive, and averse to eating. Occasionally she uttered the statement, "If thy eye offend thee, cut it out." One evening she actually broke her restraint and almost succeeded in enucleating her right eye with the thumb and forefinger of the right hand. She continued to talk incoherently, laughed a great deal in a silly manner, and made no attempt to keep her person neat and clean. After several months she improved in her general behavior, but remained withdrawn, childish and manneristic, untidy and content to sit on the floor, lost in silly phantasy, and utterly indifferent to all activity about her. Five months after her breakdown, her parents returned from Africa to visit her, but she manifested no normal interest in them; in fact, she showed no indication that she recognized them when they made their appearance in the ward.

Catatonic Type

This mental disturbance develops much more suddenly than do other forms of schizophrenia, and frequently in

Catatonic: Stupor stage
Excitement stage

individuals who are not particularly lacking in emotional development. It is characterized by an acute stupor associated with a sudden loss of all animation and a tendency to remain motionless in a stereotyped position or posture. The facial expression becomes vacant, and the skin waxy in appearance; the patient be-

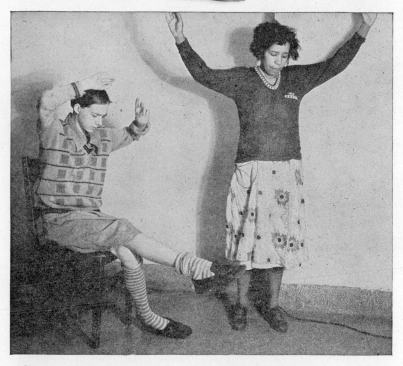

Fig. 17.—Postures and fixed positions assumed by patients with the catatonic type of schizophrenia. One individual strikes an attitude and the other attempts to do the same. This is called echopraxia.

comes mute and is apparently unable to comply with the simplest order or request. The lips are often pursed in a peculiar way; the saliva drools from the mouth; and the hands and feet may become blue and swollen because of the immobility. Such patients must be dressed.

Low B.P.   Low B.M.R.

washed, moved about by force from room to room; they are apparently insensitive to threats or to painful stimuli. If the arm is upraised to an awkward and uncom-

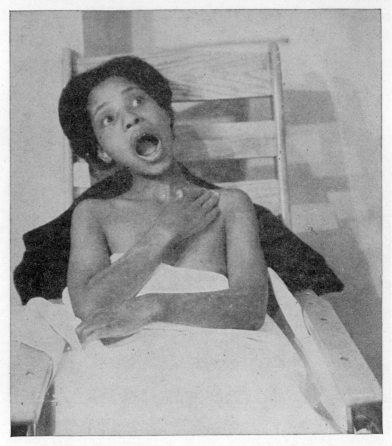

Fig. 18.—Catatonic schizophrenia, showing an unusual posture. The open mouth and the position of the arms is maintained for hours at a time.

fortable position, it may remain so for several hours. In an automatic manner the patient may imitate others (_echopraxia_) or repeat phrases in a stereotyped way (_echolalia_).

Heard things

Without warning, this passive or stupor state may give way to a violent, hateful outburst during which the patient suddenly becomes voluble, argumentative, and even homicidal. This fact every nurse must keep in mind in every case of catatonia. Such violent episodes are known as *catatonic excitement*. Suicidal frenzy may develop. The patient frequently demonstrates hallucinations at this time and may indicate from the speech content that he recalls everything which occurred during the period of immobility.

This alternation between periods of stupor and excitement gives this form of schizophrenia a distinctive quality which, in some respects, may liken it to a manic-depressive psychosis. For this reason a prolonged catatonic stupor may well be mistaken for a depressive phase as the excited state may be erroneously taken for a delirious mania. Differential diagnosis is not always easy, and it is possible that catatonia is a psychosis which in some respects is a halfway state between schizophrenia and the affective-reaction psychoses. Only when a succession of catatonic episodes eventually leads to a state of considerable dementia can one be certain that this disorder truly belongs to the schizophrenic group.

B. G., a woman 22 years old, was admitted because she refused to eat or talk and was found in her room sitting in a trancelike state in a chair, staring out of the window. The morning of the day that she was admitted she had thrown a bowl of cereal across the tray directly at her mother.

This patient has always been touchy, high strung, and inclined to have temper tantrums. She was by reputation a bookworm, had no interest in the home, demanded a great deal of attention, and thought herself to be above her family in cultural achievements. As a matter of fact, she was only a mediocre student, and most of her reading was restricted to light, shallow fiction. She belonged to a literary club and imagined herself to be one of its most brilliant members, although she rarely contributed to its regular programs.

When first employed as a stenographer, she gave her family the impression that she was indispensable to her employer. When she was among the first to be discharged as a result of the business depression some two years before her present illness, she withdrew into an aloofness during which she scarcely uttered a word to the other members of her family for a period of two months.

Her younger sister was more popular, practical, and sensible. Of her she was naturally extremely jealous. The patient, herself, was never greatly interested in the opposite sex and had had only a "platonic affair" with one of her fellow-members of the literary club. Two months before, both she and her sister took a competitive examination for a position as private secretary. The younger sister secured the position, and when she informed the patient of the results, the latter refused to believe it. Shortly thereafter she became taciturn, refused to eat and remained in the kitchen sitting near the stove with her stare fixed upon the opposite wall. She sat in this position all night, and a physician was called. He gave her a hypodermic injection, and she was taken to her room by force.

On the ward she was found standing in an awkward position with the head held slightly forward and with an inane expression on the face, the skin of which had a waxy appearance. She ignored all questions except when asked to protrude the tongue, which act she performed but failed to withdraw it back into the mouth. Her eyes were directed toward the floor. If her arm was elevated above her head, it remained in that position until the examining physicians passed on to interview other patients, at which time it was slowly dropped to a dependent position.

At meal time she resisted being escorted into the dining room. There she had to be spoon fed. Again she resisted being led out of the dining room. This resistiveness to any required conduct which is so characteristic of all types of schizophrenia is called *negativism*. At the end of the day her hands and feet were definitely cyanotic because of the fixed standing position she maintained for long intervals. She soiled her clothing and took no interest in the other patients, except to study the footwear with her downcast eyes.

She had one catatonic outburst. A manic fellow patient took special delight in tormenting her for her immobility, calling her a "dummy" and a "wooden Indian." One day, without warning, and when the manic patient was least expecting an outburst, the patient turned about, approached the other patient from behind, and yanked two handfuls of hairs out of the other's head.

The screams of the outraged patient brought nurses to the scene, to find the catatonic patient standing again in transfixed position, but with the telltale hair clenched in her hands.

Her recovery occurred just as suddenly as the illness began. One metrazol convulsion produced a dramatic change. She became accessible, answered questions intelligently, and developed a great interest in occupational therapy. Three months after admission she was quite normal. At this time she proffered the statement that she knew all along what was going on, but seemed to be "inwardly paralyzed." During the two months of her catatonic stupor she scarcely lifted her eyes, but she learned to associate the voices of the individual physicians and nurses by the appearance of their shoes. Hence, it was not surprising when she was able to identify each one as soon as she recovered from the catatonic state.

Paranoid Schizophrenia

This form of schizophrenia tends to develop at a later period of life, generally in the later twenties or the early thirties. Delusions of an absurd, illogical quality dominate the clinical picture. Behind these one always finds the usual inadequate social development and emotional lameness. Apparently the patient with paranoid schizophrenia attempts to maintain self-esteem and cover up his sense of inadequacy by explaining it away in terms of false beliefs of persecution or of grandeur; even depressive and hypochondriacal delusions are common. Not only are the delusions silly and unbelievable, but they are numerous and changeable to meet the special psychological needs as they may occur. Critical judgment is necessarily poor, and reality must be warped to fit in with the patient's own phantastic projections. Behavior is erratic, unpredictable, and even dangerous because of the paranoid condition. A good example of the silly and warped mental state of a paranoid schizophrene is the following:

I. T., a Jugoslavian male aged 32 years, was admitted because he threatened his fellow workers at the auto body plant where

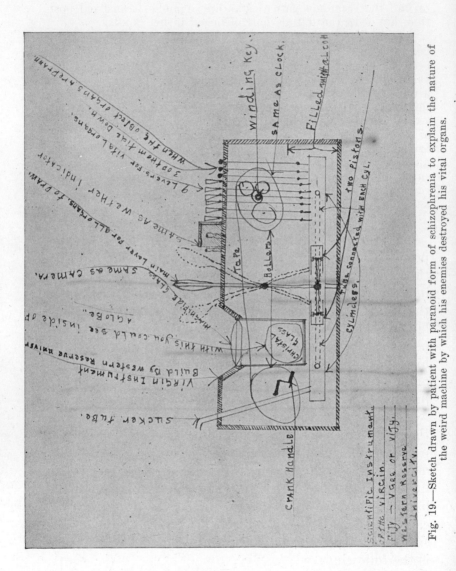

Fig. 19.—Sketch drawn by patient with paranoid form of schizophrenia to explain the nature of the weird machine by which his enemies destroyed his vital organs.

he was employed as a polisher. Little information was available about his early childhood except that he came to this country with his parents when he was 11 years old. He had a scanty night school education, spoke broken English, but was unusually interested in reading cheap magazines on popular science. He never married and had no particular social interests. Instead he had developed the habit of drinking beer and at irregular intervals was known to become quite intoxicated. He had a reputation at the shop for collecting odd bits of worthless machinery and taking them home to "invent something." His bedroom at home was filled with this useless trash with which he rarely did anything. Any attempt on the part of his mother to remove this material would bring on a loud protest and an accusation of plotting against him and his inventions.

For several months he believed his fellow workers were spying on him and were trying to steal his "invention." A woman living in the opposite end of the city was plotting to sap him of his "vital energy." This she did by developing a "sucking machine" at the local university laboratory. The machine worked by wireless and acted principally on his liver which was slowly wasting away. These details of the persecutions which he suffered he told with a perfunctory tone and with no display of affect. When asked about the mechanics of such a lethal device, with great enthusiasm he obliged by making a sketch of the machine.

Each day at ward rounds he aroused himself from his usual apathy to face the physicians and demand that the woman be imprisoned. He barricaded himself in the washroom to keep other patients out of it because they communicated with the woman through the sewer pipes. He ate ravenously, used vulgar language in the presence of the nurses, and insisted that he be allowed to work in the hospital laboratories, because he owned the institution. Occasionally, he appeared to be menacing but never actually assaulted anyone on the ward. The patient was given some thirty insulin shocks, but this treatment made little or no impression upon the mental condition.

Treatment and Nursing Care in Schizophrenia.—The majority of patients with an active schizophrenic psychosis should be treated in mental hospitals or sanatoria. The modern institution pursues a policy of active attention to the patient. The fundamental idea behind therapy is to direct the patient's interests once more toward reality. This is a difficult task, frequently unsuccessful, but even if only partially successful, it is worthwhile and gratifying. Particularly useful are occupational therapy and planned recreation activities designed to socialize the patient's interests. Moving pictures, music, games, and suitable athletics are all valuable.

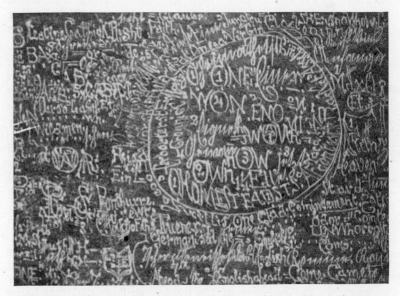

Fig. 20.—Queer hieroglyphics carved by a schizophrenic patient on a piece of slate with a nail. The symbols are undoubtedly expressive of some of the internal or autistic mental processes of the patient.

The proper care of schizophrenics demands great resourcefulness on the part of the nurse. Tact, a sympathetic attitude, and patience do much to allay apprehension and gain confidence. Insistence on proper habits respecting bodily functions and cleanliness is a start in externalizing the patient's interests. The tendency of patients to inactivity and withdrawal into phantasy can be counteracted by keeping a patient occupied with various little tasks, varying them frequently to avoid boredom.

Certain symptoms need special treatment. Schizophrenic excitements are best treated by the continuous tub or cold wet pack. Small doses of sedative drugs, preferably barbiturates, may be given to allay excitement and induce sleep. Amytal, 1½ to 3 grains, is valuable since it is not cumulative. Needless to say, drugs must be judiciously used, for there is no excuse for a toxic stupor. Restraints should not be used; they cause resentment and suspicion in the patient which may make further cooperation impossible. Isolation of the patient in a room may be necessary for a few hours or even a few days. However, since an attempt is being made at socialization, seclusion of the patient is contraindicated except for special occasions of short duration.

Catatonic stupor is a trying nursing problem. Careful attention must be paid to the bowels and bladder. The patients will retain feces for days with the formation of fecal impactions. Cathartics are to be preferred to enemas. The type of cathartic and its dosage must be determined for each patient. Mineral oil is helpful in preventing a hard dry bowel content which may form a very firm impaction. Aromatic fluidextract of cascara sagrada 2 to 4 drams (8 to 16 c.c.) and epsom salts 1 to 2 ounces (30 to 60 c.c.) are usually effective. Enemas can be used as a last resort. Olive oil retention enemas help loosen up impactions. Simple tap water or soapsuds enemas are usually as effective as those with many ingredients and elaborate formulas.

The feeding problems presented by negativistic, resistive patients can often be overcome by spoon feeding. If this is impossible, one must resort to tube feeding.

Catatonic patients should be encouraged to move about or should be given passive exercise and massage to prevent cyanosis and swelling of the extremities. A special point should be made of dressing patients with catatonic stupor in warm clothing and paying strict attention to the room temperature. The patient will often remain in a very cold room seemingly impervious to cold, only to contract pneumonia.

Special Shock Treatments of Schizophrenia.—Although schizophrenia has been treated by a great number of pharmacological agents, none of them has ever enjoyed widespread application as has insulin shock treatment. Most psychiatrists report a recovery rate with insulin treatment which is significantly greater than the recovery rate in untreated cases. The best results are obtained in early cases. During the first six months of the illness the recovery rate is highest and thereafter declines; after eighteen months complete recovery is rare although partial recovery is not infrequent. Of the various types of schizophrenia the paranoid and catatonic types respond best to insulin treatment. Although the results of insulin therapy are encouraging, yet its ultimate place in the therapy of schizophrenia is still uncertain as the permanence of recovery is unknown.

Metrazol has not given such consistently good results in schizophrenia as has insulin. Its greatest field of usefulness appears to be in the catatonic type. Besides being used alone it has been used with insulin therapy. The entire status of metrazol therapy is at present very uncertain since it has been discovered that fractures and dislocations may occur from the metrazol convulsion. The most common complications are compression fractures of the vertebrae. Since it has these undesirable side actions, metrazol should be used cautiously only in selected cases. The technique for these special therapies is given in another chapter.

References

Bleuler, Eugen: Textbook of Psychiatry, translated by A. A. Brill, New York, 1924, The Macmillan Co.

Jung, C. G.: Psychology of Dementia Praecox, translated by A. A. Brill, Nervous and Mental Disease Monographs, 1936.

Lewis, N. D. C.: Constitutional Factors in Dementia Praecox, Nervous and Mental Disease Monographs, New York.

Questions for Chapter X

Schizophrenic Reaction Types

1. Describe the schizoid temperament.
2. Briefly define schizophrenia.
3. What are the four types of schizophrenia as presented by Kraepelin? Briefly discuss each type.
4. Are these four types clear-cut and distinct or do they sometimes merge or change as the disease progresses?
5. Explain the term ''regression.''
6. Why does a catatonic patient need to be watched carefully?
7. What is the fundamental objective in nursing the schizophrene?
8. Discuss habit formation and ways to direct the patient along the road to reality.
9. What particular nursing problems do catatonic patients present and how would you meet them?
10. Briefly discuss metrazol and insulin shock therapy in schizophrenia.

*Chronic Disease — Incurable — Characterized by
(slowly progressive)   systimized delusions which have
                  as a rule a fairly logical sequence
                  but are based on false premesis.*

CHAPTER XI

PARANOID REACTION TYPES

The tendency to be sensitive, to be hurt easily, and to assign base motives to the behavior of others exists in most people to varying degrees. Apparently this disposition to blame others for one's own dissatisfactions is more prominent in those who are inherently proud but inadequate. There are thousands who go through life feeling that they are underrated, misunderstood, and abused, and whose career is blighted by bitterness, resentment, cynicism and senseless brooding over fancied wrongs and persecution. To obtain any sense of security many such individuals establish the conviction that they are hounded by persecutors and that the responsibility for their failures belongs to others. Thus the paranoid person obtains surcease from his ego torment, not only by firmly believing his own false ideas, but by convincing others that they are true.

Definition.—Paranoia is, therefore, a reaction to a state of insecurity; it is a change in personality where reason appears preserved, but is dominated by certain false convictions or beliefs. In some respects, it resembles the paranoid form of schizophrenia in that it springs from a basic personality which lacks easy and natural social adjustment. However, unlike schizophrenia, the paranoid individual is not likely to show a gradual deterioration of other mental faculties and may even conceal his mental quirks for many years before they become a matter of social concern.

Causes.—The chief causes lie in the deeper psychic structures of the individual and may be displayed even in childhood years. A desire to be praised and appreciated for minor achievements is demonstrated, and, when this is not forthcoming, there are moodiness, sulking, and a withdrawal from normal contacts. There is an abnormal craving for superiority over others. Such people are always wondering whether others talk about them and see a hidden meaning in every casual remark. An enormous and easily wounded pride is the outstanding predictive element which one finds in all people who later become paranoid. According to Freud, homosexual fixation is a common underlying factor in paranoid conditions.

Symptoms.—The signs of paranoia develop very slowly so that by the time the condition attains the proportions of a true psychosis, the individual is generally well in the adult years. A tendency to excessive brooding and daydreaming is followed by delusional notions. There is a hidden meaning in things about the patient and ideas of reference are formulated out of incidental remarks and trivial events. Slowly the patient amplifies his false ideas and distorts actual facts to fit his delusional scheme, a process known as *falsification*. The nature and complexity of his delusions depend greatly on the patient's education, his environment, and his special interests or vocation. From the persecutory stage the patient may pass into a state of grandeur, for, he argues, endless persecution by others implies envy and jealousy of his own status and it follows that he is an extraordinary person. He may present himself as a great prophet, a secret service operative, a master mind, a great inventor, or a second Christ. Thus he may appear on the streets with a long beard or in a general's uniform. Often he imagines himself abused by the courts after a minor legal affray, and proceeds to initiate further lawsuits which have no rational basis. This form of paranoia is called the *litigious* type and is merely

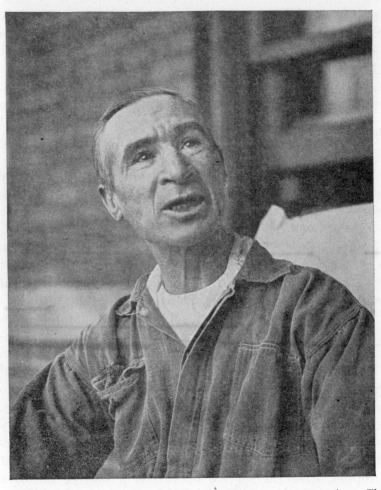

Fig. 21.—Paranoia with delusions of grandeur and persecution. The patient insisted that he was a secret service man in a high governmental position who was being detained by gangsters and refused to concede that he was a patient in the hospital.

another method whereby the patient attempts to display his superiority over others.

A fairly representative case of paranoia is demonstrated in the following case history.

A. T. was born of a white father and a mulatto mother in one of the central states. The father was a steamboat engineer and died as a result of a boiler explosion when the patient was ten years old. With his mother he lived in a decrepit part of the city where he was neither liked by the negroes nor openly received by the white children. Very early in his school years he developed a taste for mechanics, was a good student, but rather aloof and decidedly sensitive to the jibes of his schoolmates. He was thin and sallow and had very few negroid features. He spent his leisure hours in studying chemistry and physics in the city library. At the age of 15 years he had a fight in the school yard with a white boy who called his mother a "yellow nigger." After this affair he had very little to do with other young people, except with those who were interested in a city mission which he attended regularly.

His habits were good, and he was extremely esthetic in his tastes, drank no liquor, did not smoke, and showed no normal interest in the opposite sex. On graduation from high school he worked for two years in a tile factory as a shipping clerk. At this time he was awarded a scholarship and matriculated in a special college for negroes. There his social condition was not improved, for the negro students avoided him and he displayed no interest in them. At the end of two years his scholarship lapsed, and having no resources of his own he returned home and resumed his work with the same concern which previously employed him.

At the city mission during prayer meetings and on Sunday he gave long meaningless testimonials and fancied himself a promising preacher. During the summer absence of the regular minister he apparently expected to be asked to serve as a substitute. When another man was called, the patient sulked; expressed his resentment openly at the next meeting and resigned from the congregation. A few weeks later his mother passed away. He lived alone in a small upstairs flat which he was able to maintain because his mother had left a small legacy. Here he secluded himself for many weeks and emerged only once a day to buy a few groceries and a bottle of milk. His landlady, who lived below, fearing that he was

ill, climbed the stairs and knocked on the door. Receiving
no answer, she obtained a key and, on opening the patient's
room, was struck down by a baseball bat. She managed to
get to her rooms to call the police who were compelled to use
tear gas to apprehend the patient.

When admitted, he refused to give his name. He wore a
pointed beard and a loose gown resembling a monk's robe. His
demeanor was haughty. "Yes, I am an engineer—to be exact,
I'm God's own engineer. Do not concern yourself over my
real name, it has enough stigma attached to it now. No, I am
not married, but I have been tried by all the lures that women
possess. No, I don't use rotten liquor or filthy tobacco—I am
made for higher things. My enemies follow me everywhere I
go and make obscene comments about me on the walls of
public washrooms. I'm offered only menial positions so as to
keep me penniless most of the time. They put their heads
together and scheme their dastardly plans.

"See this sore [pointing to a varicose ulcer]? This is where
they inducted me with their electrical currents. That's why
I slept in a 'non-conductor' bed. I made it myself and
suspended it from insulators fixed in the ceiling. The landlady came up to destroy my devices because the bishop of
her church had ordered her to do so. The modern church is
determined to destroy me because I preach the older creeds.
[Proudly] Why should I not be hailed as the second Christ?"

The patient remained for months in the same mental condition. His attitude was patronizing, proud, and suspicious. In
other patients he showed little or no interest. He refused to
shave or have his hair cut, had no interest in occupational
therapy, and spent most of his time vacantly staring out of
the ward windows.

Prognosis and Treatment.—P a r a n o i d conditions
rarely, if ever, improve, for in most instances the disease
represents the patient's best effort in justifying his existence and placating his ego. Many individuals suffer
with this distortion of personality, but possess enough
self-control not to offend society. They exist as harmless "cranks," religious enthusiasts, or hermits. Occasionally institutional treatment with its tranquil atmosphere, where competitive tension does not exist, may do

much to alleviate the sensitivity of the paranoid person, and the major symptoms may become latent or disappear.

References

Bleuler, Eugen: Textbook of Psychiatry, translated by A. A. Brill, New York, 1924, The Macmillan Co.

Henderson and Gillespie: A Textbook of Psychiatry, Humphrey Milford, London, 1927, Oxford University Press.

Questions for Chapter XI
Paranoid Reaction Types

1. Describe the paranoid personality.
2. Differentiate between the paranoid state and the paranoid form of schizophrenia.
3. Discuss the causes of paranoia.
4. Do the symptoms develop abruptly? Give early manifestations.
5. What is falsification?
6. Why does the paranoid patient often have grandiose ideas?
7. What is the usual prognosis in paranoia? What reason can you give for this?
8. Would you try to convince a paranoid patient that his delusions are false?
9. What are some of the most common delusions expressed by the paranoid person?
10. What is litigious paranoia?

CHAPTER XII — *organic psychoses*

REACTION TYPES WITH SOMATIC DISEASE—
SYMPTOMATIC PSYCHOSES

The human brain is sensitive to a wide range of poisons and reacts with varying degrees of organic derangement. As a highly specialized organ, it requires an unfailing amount of oxygen and has an elaborate blood supply which cannot be seriously disturbed without creating havoc. Like other organs of the body, the brain suffers whenever there is some systemic disease which elaborates poisons or which impairs circulation. Whenever the brain function is affected as a result of some general physical disease, the mental condition is known as a *symptomatic* psychosis.

While symptomatic psychoses are not particularly frequent, the causes are of many kinds. The most common mental reaction is a delirious state. The delirium may be mild or severe. It implies some degree of clouding of consciousness, a tendency to tremor and to fumbling movements of the hands and fingers, and in the severe forms there are vivid hallucinations of sight. The delirious patient may see terrifying images of animals, human faces, dancing objects, or merely flashes of light. There may also be hallucinations of touch, as if insects were crawling over the body. If the patient recovers from a delirium, he generally fails to recall any events which occurred during the period of confusion.

The nurse should remember that delirium may be of fleeting occurrence. It may last but a few minutes to be followed by a lucid period and frequently may be manifested by merely a frightened look or a muttering of a few unintelligible words. It is important that such a delirium be detected, for it may play an important part in establishing a prognosis. Except in children, the appearance of delirium generally indicates a grave physical state, no matter what the fundamental cause may be. Old people are particularly prone to a delirious state in the presence of cardiac failure.

Psychoses With Acute Infectious Diseases

Very young children, men who are chronic alcoholics, and old people develop delirium very quickly if an infection is severe and the fever is very high. It is most frequently noted in lobar pneumonia, cerebrospinal and tuberculous meningitis, influenza, scarlet fever, malaria, and typhoid fever. Delirium is more likely to occur at night. If a patient with a high fever becomes restless, tires easily, and seems to have difficulty in grasping simple statements, one should be on guard and suspect an impending delirious state. The patient wanders in speech content, seems dreamy, dazed, and apprehensive. There may be fumbling with the bedclothes, and the patient generally looks about him in a bewildered manner. Persons are not clearly recognized, or the patient may look at his visitors with apparently unseeing eyes. If the delirium deepens into deep stupor or coma, the condition is undeniably grave.

In some acute infections, such as measles, somnolence is very common and is not particularly significant. Occasionally the delirium of an acute infection may include agitation and sudden irritability. The patient may even climb out of bed and walk about in a confused manner. This frequently occurs in the delirium of typhoid fever.

Psychoses With Acute Chorea

Chorea is closely associated with acute rheumatic fever and is now recognized as a true brain disease, although the exact toxic factor is unknown. Apart from the jerky, involuntary movements which are so characteristic of the disease, there may be pronounced mental symptoms. The child with chorea is not only restless but often becomes irritable, sensitive and quarrelsome; he has insomnia and frequent nightmares. Hysterical outbursts are easily provoked, and in severe cases there may be a true delirium.

Cardiac Psychoses

This term is applied strictly to those mental states induced by failing circulation by reason of cardiac deficiency alone, and not to the confusion of elderly people who have, in addition, some form of cerebral sclerosis. Such mental confusion may be encountered in heart block where the pulse is very slow, in mitral stenosis where the pulse is too small and threadlike, and in acute cardiac conditions in younger people where the heart muscle has been badly damaged by infections and poisons. The delirium in these cases is generally mild and fleeting. The patient becomes irritable, apprehensive and occasionally excited, suspicious, and even combative. Objects and persons are misidentified, and true hallucinations may occur although these are not prominent.

Puerperal Psychoses

During the eight weeks following childbirth, a number of women become acutely psychotic and develop a true delirium. There may or may not be a fever associated with this condition. While the puerperal delirium itself is not particularly significant, it generally leads to more serious protracted mental disorders of the manic-depressive or schizophrenic types.

Treatment of Symptomatic Psychoses.—It is obvious that the treatment of symptomatic delirium is essentially the treatment of the infection or circulatory defect which is the disturbing factor. In acute infections, cold wet packs have a markedly beneficial effect on delirious states. Bed rest and absolute seclusion from any extraneous excitement are essential. To this end such sedatives as chloral hydrate or paraldehyde are recommended. Delirium in the presence of very high fever may be abated by giving sodium salicylate or aspirin in 10 grain doses three times a day. Because delirium may be an expression of vitamin deficiency, the administration of 10 to 50 mg. of vitamin B_1 daily by the intravenous or the hypodermic route frequently does more than anything else to terminate the psychosis.

Nursing Care of Delirious Patients.—Irrespective of the cause, the delirious patient is critically ill and requires diligent bedside supervision. The patient should be secluded from others in a quiet, darkened room, and visitors should be limited to the members of the family. No restraint is necessary unless the patient is left alone. The hands should never be tightly secured by wrist cuffs, for the excessive movements may cause abrasion of the forearms.

Applying cold compresses to the head serves to reduce the excitement and mental confusion. A cool sponge bath in bed very frequently will induce normal and refreshing sleep. The skin is usually dry and hot and should be closely watched for abrasions and pressure spots. Cold cream to the lips prevents fissuring; the mouth and tongue should be cleansed several times a day.

Feeding should begin with high caloric fluids, and, as rapidly as the patient can tolerate it, semisolid and solid foods are added. Water in ample quantities should be given at frequent intervals, particularly if the fever is constant and dehydration is present.

Every effort is to be made to insure free elimination, and, as in every helpless and bedridden patient, the bladder should be guarded against distention.

All procedures and treatments are carried out at one time so far as it is possible. It is important to keep in mind that the patient should be subjected to a minimum amount of stimulation and that rest is a most essential part of the management of a patient who is toxic, restless, and delirious.

The recovery from any systemic condition which causes delirium is necessarily slow. Relapses into a confusional state are not at all uncommon. For a long period after the acute illness there remains easy mental and physical fatigue which contraindicates any excessive exercise or mental concentration. Some simple form of occupational therapy can be prescribed as soon as the patient expresses a desire to do it, but this should be allowed for only short periods. As physical strength is regained, walking in the open air is recommended to reestablish muscular coordination and self-confidence.

Reference

Noyes, Arthur: Modern Clinical Psychiatry, ed. 2, Philadelphia, 1939, W. B. Saunders Co.

Questions for Chapter XII

Reaction Types With Somatic Disease—Symptomatic Psychoses

1. What is the cause of a symptomatic psychosis?
2. What symptoms are associated with a delirium?
3. Why is it important to note and report fleeting delirious states?
4. What are the signs of an impending delirious state?
5. Name four physical diseases which might be accompanied by a psychosis.
6. What is the obvious treatment for a symptomatic psychosis?
7. Discuss the nursing care of delirious patients, covering the following points: feeding; how to make the patient comfortable; necessity of close supervision; avoidance of distressing stimuli.

CHAPTER XIII

REACTION TYPES WITH SOMATIC DISEASE—PSYCHOSES WITH ENDOCRINE DISEASE

The influence of endocrine disturbance as a specific and primary cause of mental disease has been overrated. Increasing knowledge of the function of the ductless glands has led to much speculation as to the interrelationship of their secretions and the central nervous system. Some interesting findings have been made, particularly in reference to the function of the pituitary gland and its intimate connection with the vegetative centers of the brain in the region of the third ventricle. The intriguing idea that the endocrine glands dictate the nature of one's personality has no sound scientific basis.

It is true, however, that in early life endocrine deficiencies definitely distort and retard mental and emotional development. Mental retardation is the outstanding psychic feature of these "juvenile" disturbances. All of them are complex endocrine problems, and only a few are clearly understood.

Froehlich's Syndrome

This is primarily a defect in the pituitary gland, involving both the anterior and posterior lobes. There is poor development of bone growth and of the sexual organs—a condition called infantilism. The body retains the chubby proportions of the infant. In addition, the child may have an abnormal thirst and an increased output of urine. Retardation of intellect is the rule, but a few show superior intelligence. Emotional instability and hysteria are usually displayed.

163

Cretinism

Cretinism is due to congenital deficiency of thyroid function. The body is dwarfed, the skin is dry, the lids are swollen. Mental deficiency ranges from idiocy to borderline feeblemindedness. The general appearance is that of a coarse-faced, short, stocky, stupid-looking child. If treatment is instituted early enough with one grain of thyroid extract three times daily, the effects are frequently short of miraculous.

Psychoses With Hyperthyroidism

In spite of the fact that almost all patients with hyperthyroidism are extremely tense, tremorous, and emotionally unstable, relatively few of them develop a true psychosis. When a mental disease actually appears in connection with toxic goiter, it is not a specific or typical reaction. It can be admitted, however, that the underlying personality of one who has hyperthyroidism is rather characteristic. Back of the glandular disease is a sensitive, high-strung, quick-acting individual whose feelings about every problem are very intense, whose sense of security is easily disturbed.

The "nervousness" of hyperthyroidism includes the well-known tremor, the rapid heart rate, excessive sweating, reflex excitement, great sensitivity to noise, insomnia, and general apprehensiveness. What true psychosis may be superimposed depends upon the basic personality of the patient. This may be manic excitement, agitation, a paranoid state, or a delirium-like confusion with auditory and visual hallucinations.

A good example of how the thyroid principle may bring forth a psychosis is presented in the following story:

A. T., an obese woman aged 44 years, was admitted to the Psychopathic Hospital with all the signs of mania. She was by nature a jolly, lively woman who was fond of food and had gradually taken on so much weight that she became the butt of many jokes and much raillery. She weighed 225 pounds. She determined to take "reducing tablets," and for a period of three weeks consumed some 10 to 15 grains of thyroid extract daily. Ten days before admission she became very nervous, suffered with tachycardia, became short of breath, could not sleep, and had a mild fever. She paced the floor all night, had no appetite, and complained of a severe frontal headache. Two days before admission she became visually hallucinated; there were fish floating about her. She cried frequently and heard voices under the bed. She screamed so loudly and was so violently resistive that commitment was necessary.

Examination disclosed the symptoms of extreme hyperthyroidism. She talked with a flight of ideas, repeated questions, was incoherent, disoriented and hallucinated. The pulse rate was over 160 per minute, the temperature 102° F. The tongue and lips were very dry; the skin was moist and hung in large folds where she had lost a great deal of adipose tissue. There was a coarse tremor of all extremities.

The mania continued for four weeks; after this she was able to cooperate in a basal metabolism test, the reading being +64 per cent. During the next three weeks she was moderately depressed, although the metabolic rate was still +30. After ten weeks she was entirely normal except for a fine tremor of the hands. Her weight on discharge was 155 pounds.

Her "thyroid" psychosis was apparently a delirious mania. On looking into her past history, however, it was revealed that some eighteen years before, she had suffered with a similar attack of mania which occurred immediately after childbirth. Apparently the thyroid poisoning acted merely as an immediate exciting factor in producing a mental disease to which she was constitutionally disposed.

Psychosis of Myxedema

This occurs in women and is probably the only specific mental disease produced by glandular deficiency. It was accurately described by Gull in 1877. Its symptoms are fairly constant. When thyroid deficiency occurs in adult life, mental sluggishness and physical torpor are certain to follow. The patient becomes sleepy, slow in thought and action, shows memory defects, and may become paranoid and irritable. Diagnosis is rarely difficult, for

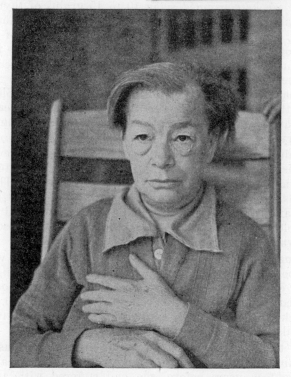

Fig. 22.—A depressed patient showing the puffy face and hands of a severe hypothyroidism or myxedema. Under appropriate treatment the mental and physical condition was radically improved.

with these mental signs, the physical features are unmistakable. The face and hands become puffy, there may be edema of the feet, the skin is dry, the hair is thin, the blood pressure is low, and the heart action is feeble. In extreme cases the patient becomes so weak that she is unable to walk. The spinal fluid may show a marked increase in protein. The mental and physical signs are best illustrated by a record of the following case:

S. T., a woman 52 years of age, had been chair-ridden for nearly two years. She was hospitalized because she refused to eat and because she believed she was being poisoned by her relatives.

On examination she was found to be in an extremely weakened condition, being unable to stand without support. She had enormous pouches under both eyes; the skin was dry and rough; both hands were puffy. The temperature was 96.2° F., the pulse was 62, and the systolic blood pressure was 88 mm. The heart was enlarged. The spinal fluid protein was increased. Basal metabolism was –32 per cent. All tendon reflexes were sluggish or absent.

Mentally she was very torpid. Answers were slow and incomplete. Her memory for recent events was poor. She admitted that she ate poorly because she believed her food was being poisoned. She groped for words when attempting to express herself and cried frequently when she appeared unable to gather her thoughts to answer questions.

It required over six weeks of heavy medication with thyroid extract, 5 grains twice a day, before she became more alert and cooperative. Her blood pressure rose to normal, the pulse mounted to 70, and the metabolic rate was –10 per cent. Gradually appetite returned, and her delusions in reference to poisoning were discarded. She was discharged with the admonition that she must continue taking 3 grains of thyroid daily for an indefinite time.

Psychosis With Acromegaly

This glandular disease, which is due to a tumor of the pituitary, not only produces a monstrous distortion of the cranial bones and a coarseness of the facial expression, but may lead in many cases to a chronic mental deterioration. The patient becomes mentally sluggish, forgetful, moody and not infrequently suspicious and paranoid. A few instances of mania have been reported.

Psychoses With Other Glandular Diseases

Mental symptoms may be attributed directly or indirectly to other endocrine disorders, but these are not so frequent as to merit anything more than a passing statement. In the adrenal deficiency of Addison's disease there may be mental depression and irritability. In parathyroid disease where tetany occurs, rare instances of confusion and hallucinosis with true convulsions have been reported. Diabetic patients are said to have mental symptoms occasionally which can be conditioned by the disease, but too many other factors are involved to make this a clear clinical picture.

References

Chadwick, Mary: The Psychological Effects of Menstruation, New York, 1932, Nervous and Mental Disease Publishing Co.
Hoskins, R. G.: The Tides of Life, New York, 1933, W. W. Norton & Co.

Questions for Chapter XIII

Psychoses With Endocrine Disease

1. Is the personality dominated by the endocrine glands? Discuss this question.
2. Describe the symptoms of (a) Froehlich's syndrome, (b) cretinism.
3. What is the standard treatment for cretinism?
4. Are psychoses with hyperthyroidism of frequent occurrence?
5. Upon what does the type of psychosis depend?
6. What is the cause of myxedema? Name the mental and physical symptoms. What is the specific treatment?
7. What is acromegaly? What are the cause and possible mental symptoms?
8. Name other glandular diseases with which psychoses may be associated.

Diabetes: Hopeless attitude

CHAPTER XIV

DELIRIOUS REACTION TYPES—ALCOHOLIC. PSYCHOSES *Exogenous - Toxic reactive*

Causes.—There has always been a great variety of opinions expressed about the use and the effect of alcohol, both as a moral and physiological issue. As yet no concerted agreement has been reached as to how much alcohol can be consumed without harmful effect. In general, those individuals who take alcohol to excess do so because they are unhappy, distraught, and maladjusted, and because alcohol furnishes them a temporary release from the stresses of living. Most alcoholics are fundamentally unstable, sensitive, self-indulgent people, and probably many of them are suffering with a poorly developed sexuality. Drink offers not only a surcease from their feelings of inferiority, but provides an occasion for conviviality and sympathy, and engenders a false sense of ease and security. Inhibitions are weakened, and repressed desires may be freely expressed. In this manner ethical and moral sense is blunted, the drinker living at a level of responsibility where high social adaptation is no longer possible. Moreover, alcohol serves to release latent or hidden dispositions to mental disease. Its effects are not uniform and may bring to the surface many different types of reaction, some of these apparently being determined by racial, social and temperamental factors which naturally vary with each individual.

While the general use of alcohol and ordinary drunkenness is a complex and immense social problem, it is the alcoholic psychosis with which the doctor and the nurse are immediately concerned. Alcoholic psychoses contribute, at the present time, between 10 and 15 per cent of the first admissions to hospitals for mental disease in the United States. During the World War this percentage was sharply reduced and rose but very slowly during the prohibition era. Mental diseases due to alcohol are predominantly found in men.

Types of Alcoholic Psychoses.—Mental diseases due to alcohol may be conveniently divided into two classes. The *acute reactions,* which consist essentially of confusion, excitement, and delirium, are of relatively short duration and do not cause a profound and permanent change in the personality. The most common of these, acute reactions are (1 pathological intoxication, (2) delirium tremens, and (3) acute alcoholic hallucinosis. The *chronic reactions,* on the other hand, imply some degree of brain degeneration and show various defects in memory and emotional control with marked personality changes which are generally permanent. These chronic states include (1) Korsakow's psychosis, (2) alcoholic paranoia, and (3) alcoholic dementia or deterioration.

Pathological Intoxication

Certain people with an unstable, hysterical temperament or those suffering with epilepsy are likely to react to even moderate amounts of alcohol with sudden and violent outbursts of mental confusion, the so-called *mania à potu.* The patient suddenly becomes hallucinated and disoriented; he may become homicidal and run about the streets in mad anxiety. This is usually followed by a period of deep sleep; and on awakening, the individual has no recollection of what has occurred.

Delirium Tremens

This is perhaps the most familiar of all the acute alcoholic mental states. It usually follows a heavy alcoholic debauch but may occur during a period of abstinence. In the latter instance a slight trauma, particularly to the head, may be the precipitating factor. It is probably true that delirium tremens is more likely to develop if the individual partakes of little food for a considerable interval and lives on alcohol alone.

The delirium is preceded by loss of appetite, restlessness, and insomnia. Slight noises cause the patient to jerk with fear, and moving objects lead to great excitement and agitation. Gradually consciousness becomes badly clouded, friends are no longer recognized, and designs in the wallpaper appear as insects or crawling animals. The patient becomes terrified and crawls across the bed or the floor to escape gruesome animals. Imaginary threads are picked off the bedclothing and creeping insects are felt and seen on the skin. Occasionally the delirious patient may give expression to a pathetic, half-hearted smile as if he were amused by his visual experiences. Only rarely does the patient show a euphoria rather than a state of fear. There is a ceaseless fumbling and picking movement of the fingers and hands; the face has an anxious or terrified expression; and the eyes are bloodshot. The skin is moist with perspiration; the tongue and the lips are tremorous. The pulse is rapid and weak, and there is always some elevation of temperature.

The death rate in delirium tremens is high: 10 to 15 per cent of the patients die with heart failure or bronchopneumonia as the most frequent fatal complication. Autopsy reveals a "wet brain" due to edema.

The following history furnishes a typical case report:

M. M., male, age 29 years, was admitted to the Psychopathic Ward from a boardinghouse where he was found in delirium tremens. He was unmarried, worked intermittently as a dock laborer, and shared his room with a fellow worker with whom he was accustomed to drink at a nearby saloon. He had been drinking excessively for some three weeks. The day before admission he was excitable and quarrelsome, and accused his roommate of throwing sand down his neck. During the night he mumbled to himself, rolled about, and fell out of bed. He claimed a dozen dogs were looking in at the window. Toward morning he was stuporous, shaky, and incoherent.

On admission he was put to bed where he crawled about with a terrified expression on his face. Restraint was necessary. He picked incessantly at his wrist cuffs and at the bedclothes. He was able to mumble his name, but little more. During short lucid moments he admitted sheepishly that he had been drinking too much and asked for another "shot." He insisted that he saw leering faces on the walls and that there was a leopard under the bed. He was dehydrated, feverish, the eyes were bloodshot, and his gaze shifted constantly from one corner of the room to another.

Twelve days after admission his sensorium cleared. He was able to give a clear account of his past, but remembered nothing of the first ten days of his hospital experience. In fact, he was greatly puzzled to find himself in a hospital bed and inquired into the identity of the institution.

Acute Alcoholic Hallucinosis

There is some question as to whether this terrifying psychosis is essentially alcoholic. By some it is regarded as a primary personality disorder which is simply brought to the surface by alcoholic indulgence. In this condition consciousness remains clear except that the patient suddenly hears voices discussing his innermost private weaknesses, particularly those of a sexual nature. His misdemeanors and deficiencies are itemized, after which inventory a suitable punishment is proposed. He may hear the clanking of chains, the sharpening of knives, or the firing of pistols, all approaching in a threatening fashion. This terrifies the patient, and frequently in his agony he makes a half-hearted attempt at suicide with whatever is at hand or runs screaming for help to the nearest police station. This hallucinosis may remain for several days or even weeks during which time the patient is also somewhat depressed, but otherwise well-oriented and coherent. Upon recovery he recalls with a feeling of shame all his abnormal experiences and is generally able to appreciate that his troubles are due to excessive drinking.

A good example of the personality which underlies this condition and the manner in which alcoholic hallucinosis accentuates the deficiences in character is given herewith:

A. T., a machinist by trade, 32 years old, was regarded as a backward individual in a social sense, living quietly with an aged mother and having no particular pleasures except an occasional Saturday night debauch. He was never easy in the presence of the opposite sex but was greatly dependent upon his mother. One Saturday night he returned home in a fairly well intoxicated state and was put to bed with considerable difficulty. Early the next morning he aroused his mother from sleep by crying "Murder!" "Help me!" She burst into his room to find him running about holding a hammer, with which he was pounding at his right temple. Her entreaties to calm himself only maddened him the more. "They accuse me of assaulting my little niece and call me a dirty dog. Listen to them—I know they'll get me if I don't kill myself first." Abruptly he ran for a door at the end of the hall and jumped through the sash, glass and all, to a snow-covered lawn next door. In nightclothes and without shoes he ran for several blocks in sheer terror until seized by a policeman who conducted him by wagon to the police ward.

In the hospital he appeared dejected and apathetic; he avoided contact with other patients. Due to exposure he had frostbite of several toes and for several weeks was confined to bed. At night he continued to hear the voices of his tormentors. The voices promised to dismember him because he was a rapist. He ate poorly but was otherwise submissive and cooperative. Three weeks after admission, there was no evidence of hallucinosis; the patient was grateful, and his insight was good. He recalled all his harrowing experiences and admitted that he was probably "crazy from liquor."

Treatment of Acute Alcoholic Psychoses.—It is almost needless to point out that in all acute intoxications associated with mental upset, alcohol must be withdrawn at once. The practice of "tapering off" alcoholics with small doses of whiskey has no justifiable basis. The patient should be put to bed, and, if restraint is necessary, it should be applied as loosely as possible to prevent senseless struggling and chafing of the skin. The continuous bath is frequently recommended, but with a terrified or hallucinated patient this procedure may be extremely exhaustive and any advantage gained may be offset by the excitement so induced. The same may be said of the wet pack. Paraldehyde in 3 or 4 teaspoonful doses two or three times a day is the sedative preferred by most physicians. A spinal puncture whereby pressure within the cranium can be reduced by withdrawing 25 to 50 c.c. of the fluid may be a very beneficial procedure. Fluids should be administered liberally. Intravenous hypertonic glucose to reduce the fluid content of the brain is of questionable value.

Probably most potent a relieving measure is the intravenous or intramuscular injection of crystalline vitamin B_1 or thiamine, for it is now appreciated that a major cause of delirium tremens is an inadequate intake of this vitamin principle. It is believed that 25 to 50 mg. of thiamine chloride intravenously daily for four or five days definitely shortens the period of delirium, abates the restlessness, and promotes normal rest and sleep.

Crude liver, 2 to 4 c.c. by subcutaneous injection appears to have the same beneficial effect. Where cardiac damage is suspected, a digitalis preparation should also be given in average doses. Alkalis, such as 10 to 15 gr. of sodium bicarbonate three times daily, are of value to offset the tendency to acidosis.

Probably the most sensible and efficacious therapy is adequate feeding with a high caloric diet. Brewers' yeast is a simple and economic method of assuring ample intake of vitamin B_1. Recovery from a typical delirium

Dypsomania — Periodical drinkers — Have morbid desire to get liquor & don't want to break away from alcohol.

tremens may be abrupt, but rest and good food are essential to prevent early relapse and to build up the general resistance of the patient.

Korsakow's Psychosis

In some respects this interesting form of alcoholism, first described by Korsakow in 1887, is an acute alcoholic reaction, but, because it often leaves in its wake a certain degree of personality change and blunting of intellectual capacity, it should be regarded as evidence of brain damage. In this condition the patient may appear to be delirious, but more accurately the picture is one of memory defect which is concealed by falsification. *(confabulation)* The patient has a memory gap for recent events and regales the listener with fanciful tales which apparently fill in such loss of memory. In addition, there is a peripheral neuritis with tingling of the extremities or in severe cases there may be wrist and foot drop.

Characteristically, there are pronounced changes in the brain cells as well as degenerative disease of the peripheral nerves. All these disturbances are definitely due to a deficiency of vitamin B₁. Treatment with thiamine, brewers' yeast, and a vitamin-rich diet of milk, fruit, and meat generally restores the patient to nearly normal physical and mental health. However, as mentioned before, there remain minor impairments of memory, emotional control, and ethical behavior which mark the individual as a chronic alcoholic. *Confabulation — if parts of story forgotten, parts are then substituted, so story sounds complete.*

Alcoholic Paranoia

As in other paranoid conditions this psychosis actually arises out of certain inadequacies of the personality, particularly in the sexual sphere. Men and women who develop this psychosis are by nature stubborn, suspicious, and jealous people. The innate fear of impotence, particularly acute in the years of middle life, is projected as an abnormal distrust of the mate, and delusions of jealousy and infidelity are the most common mental symptoms. These delusions are tenaciously cherished and supported by the most trivial and silly arguments. Men who pride themselves on their sexual prowess are particularly prone to this mental obsession and may go to extremes to prove their suspicions and sustain their delusions. In a drunken rage of jealousy they may slay their wives. Deterioration in other spheres of intellect may not be great, and in ordinary contact men with alcoholic paranoia frequently give one the impression that they are normal husbands who have been betrayed by unfaithful wives. An example of this form of alcoholic deterioration is presented in the following case study.

M. F., aged 49 years, a flour salesman, had been suspicious of his wife for several years. His sexual demands had become excessive, but apparently his potency was declining. He had been drinking regularly but rarely became intoxicated. Each night he locked the bedroom door, nailed the windows shut, and slept with a revolver within reach. In spite of all these precautions he was convinced that after he fell asleep, his wife anesthetized him with "dope" and crept out of the room to meet her paramour.

One morning he saw his wife emerging from an old barn in the rear of the house, where she had been gathering eggs. Seeing a few wisps of straw or hay on her back, he proceeded to get a fork and to look for the lover in the hayloft. He was arrested by the sheriff.

After admission to the hospital he appeared well-mannered, coherent and well-oriented. He made no mention of his delusions but merely stated that he had "a little family trouble." After a few days he was released because his neighbors, who knew nothing of his domestic affairs, insisted that he was normal. A few weeks later he was readmitted because he accused a neighboring barber of being his wife's lover and threatened him with a gun. At this time he freely expressed his ideas of infidelity and told a rather convincing story. These delusions he maintained for many months, although for short periods he expressed the opinion that he may have been in error. It was the opinion of the attending psychiatrists that the outlook for recovery was poor.

Alcoholic Deterioration

This is the end result of prolonged and excessive drinking and is essentially a chronic dementia. The onset is gradual, and a slow personality change occurs which becomes more evident to the family than it does on the street or in the shop. This phase of the disease is aptly described by the term "house devil and street angel." The patient inevitably becomes coarsened and impulsive in behavior, and moral sense is low. The patient lacks perseverance, becomes maudlin, and careless as to appearance. He will not brook any criticism of his drinking, becoming touchy and irritable. He indulges in shallow rationalizations to explain away his drinking. There is a certain guile and superficial poise in contacts with outsiders and a fawning respect for authority, but at home the chronic alcoholic is a petty tyrant whose conduct in the presence of his wife and children is vile and shameless. It is needless to say that his capacity for work suffers greatly and that he not only neglects his family but becomes dependent upon them for support. Chronic alcoholic degeneration represents one of the most common and bitter social tragedies which blights family life. Its malignant influence may extend to many innocent individuals, particularly the children, in whom it may leave a deep psychological mark.

Treatment of Chronic Alcoholism.—Every alcoholic drinks for a reason and that reason is fundamentally an inability to adjust to certain demands of normal living or some basic defect in personality. Occasionally this disorder can be rectified, and the necessity for alcohol is no longer present. Hence, the primary treatment of the alcoholic is to aid the patient in meeting life's responsibilities without utilizing alcohol as an escape mechanism. This generally means a long period of re-education which is best done in an institution. Occupational therapy has a special value.

Obviously if deterioration is well established, such measures will bear little fruit, for one whose habit of drinking is of long standing may deny it, but he actually does not want to be free of his craving. In such cases, commitment to an institution for an indefinite time is the only solution, for society must be protected from one whose mental faculties are so badly blunted and who is such a menace and burden to his family.

References

Carroll, Robert S.: What Price Alcohol? New York, 1941, The Macmillan Co.

Emerson, Haven (editor): Alcohol and Man, New York, 1935, The Macmillan Co.

King, Marian: The Revcovery of Myself, New Haven, 1931, Yale University Press.

Seabrook, Wm.: Asylum, New York, 1935, Harcourt, Brace & Co.

Strecker and Chambers: Alcohol, One Man's Meat, New York, 1938, The Macmillan Co.

Questions for Chapter XIV

Delirious Reaction Types—Alcoholic Psychoses

1. Give some reasons for excessive drinking.
2. Distinguish between acute and chronic alcoholic reactions.
3. Describe an attack of delirium tremens.
4. What are zooscopic hallucinations?
5. What are the symptoms of acute alcoholic hallucinosis?
6. What physical disease must you guard against in acute alcoholic psychoses?
7. Deficiency of what vitamin principle is common in alcoholic psychoses?
8. Describe a case of Korsakow's psychosis.
9. What is the outstanding symptom of alcoholic paranoia?
10. Is it possible that brain changes may take place owing to alcoholic excess?
11. Describe the personality in chronic alcoholic deterioration.

CHAPTER XV

DELIRIOUS REACTION TYPES—PSYCHOSES DUE TO DRUGS

There are probably many poisons which, when taken internally, cause abnormal mental reactions. Not all of them are taken intentionally; some may be absorbed slowly without the knowledge of the individual. Examples of this form of poisoning are lead and manganese, both of which are encountered in industry. The inhalation of exhaust fumes from automobile engines, which contain carbon monoxide, likewise act as a toxin on brain tissue. These chemical substances in small doses cause fatigue, irritability, dizziness and headache. When large amounts are absorbed or when these poisons slowly accumulate, delirium, loss of memory, and stupor may result. A chronic condition resembling parkinsonism with tremor and spasticity also results from absorption of these substances.

Far more important and more common are the mental disorders caused by the intentional and habitual use of drugs which deaden the senses, such as morphine, bromides, and the barbituric acid sedatives.

Morphine Addiction

The habitual use of morphine is generally found in individuals who are unstable, weak of will, and lacking in the capacity to face reality. Very few of them have actually acquired the habit from thoughtless overmedication by a physician, although many addicts claim this to be the cause of their affliction. Morphine addicts are notorious liars for the reason that they desire to con-

179

ceal the habit from others and must resort to every form
of deceit and subterfuge to obtain the drug through illegal channels.

The victim of morphinism must live close to his source
of supply, which means that he is compelled to associate

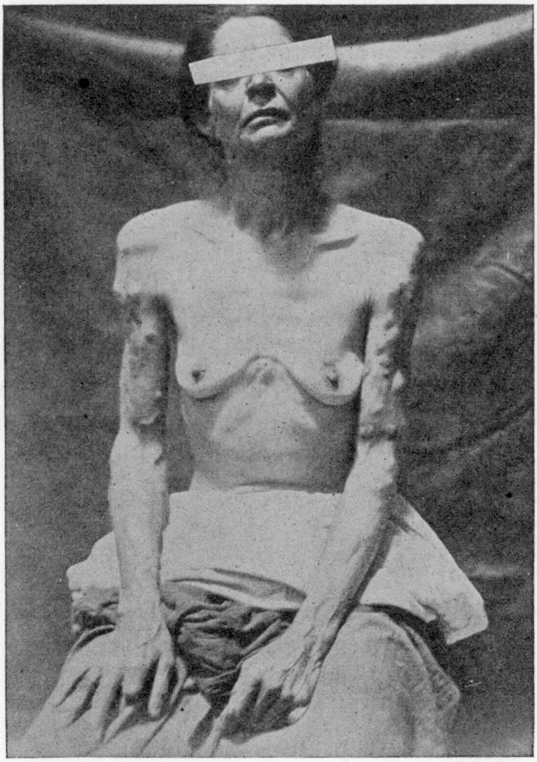

Fig. 23.—Chronic morphine addiction. The swellings on the arms are due
to multiple abscesses caused by unsterilized hypodermic injections.

with others of the same psychopathic stripe. The drug
produces a temporary state of well-being, troubles appear to be trifling and remote, and there is a comfortable
sense of complete relaxation. Ever-increasing amounts
are necessary to produce this exhilaration so that the

chronic morphine addict may require as much as 15 to 20 grains daily. Moreover, when the effects wear off and insufficient amounts are not immediately available, certain *withdrawal symptoms* promptly appear. The eyes become suffused with tears; sneezing, coryza, yawning, great irritability, and restlessness become quickly evident. Within twenty-four hours this is followed by abdominal cramps, vomiting, and diarrhea. To these distressing symptoms are added headache, sweating, and pains in the muscles and joints of the lower extremities. Finally, on the third day of abstinence the nervous irritability is so pronounced that the patient becomes hysterical, noisy, and threatening, he frequently throws and destroys objects within his reach. Within a week, however, all these painful withdrawal reactions disappear.

Most addicts are undernourished, either because they have anorexia or because they have insufficient funds to purchase enough food. Morphine, like alcohol, impairs judgment and destroys the social value of its victim. Contrary to general opinion, the morphine addict is not a fiend, or a criminal; he is, in fact, a coward who shrinks from authority and commits a minor offense only to obtain money to buy the drug. He is usually a timid, sallow, tremorous individual who only becomes assertive when he has had an injection of morphine. Whenever he obtains an adequate dose, he may expose his addiction with an abnormal euphoria and contentment or even a sleepy languor. The pupils may show a telltale "pinpoint" constriction, and in most instances the arms and thighs are scarred or pigmented by the hypodermic needle.

Treatment of Morphinism.—It is absolutely necessary to treat the morphine addict in a closed institution in order to prevent the concealed continuance of the habit. Gradual withdrawal of the drug with palliative treatment of the withdrawal symptoms is probably the most effective measure. On the first day the patient should receive about 2 or 3 grains, which is approximately the amount necessary to allay the worst of the withdrawal pains. On the second and third days the dose is reduced to 1 grain, giving ¼ grain every four hours. On the fourth day ⅙ grain of morphine is allowed four times a day; on the fifth day this is reduced to ⅛ grain; a hypodermic of sterile water is injected on the day following. The patient should not be informed as to the dosage given at any time.

Bismuth subcarbonate or sodium bicarbonate in 15 grain doses three times a day and a saline cathartic before breakfast are given to control the diarrhea and nausea. Paraldehyde in doses of 15 c.c. by rectum is recommended for its sedative effect upon the restlessness and irritability. A hot sitz bath may do much to relieve the cramping pains in the joints and muscles. If the withdrawal symptoms are bad and collapse is imminent, it is often necessary to resume the use of morphine. Addicts who are weakened by old age or incurable organic disease, particularly in the presence of cardiac deficiency, should be maintained indefinitely on morphine and reduction treatment should be avoided.

Prognosis.—With a few notable exceptions, most victims of morphine addiction rapidly relapse after reduction treatment. Sooner or later they gravitate into the old habit of seeking their old associations, of visiting old haunts, and of finding life more tolerable by resuming the old addiction and the artificial sense of security it affords.

Psychoses Due to Bromides

Bromides are universally dispensed in the form of proprietary drugs and can be purchased freely and without prescription. They are taken indiscriminately by nervous individuals, by alcoholics, and by persons for the treatment of insomnia. Large doses of this drug are used in the control of epilepsy. Bromides gradually accumulate, and, when the blood bromide mounts to 150 mg. per 100 c.c., intoxication signs are almost certain to develop. Old people with arteriosclerosis are particularly susceptible to bromide poisoning. The first signs of intoxication are fatigue, slurred speech, slowness of response, and memory defect. Very soon there develops a mental depression, the patient becomes morose, cries on little provocation, is tremorous, and stumbles about with an unsteady gait. In extreme cases this condition progresses to a true delirium with hallucinations and loss of memory which are accompanied by falsifications, not unlike a Korsakow's alcoholic psychosis.

Treatment of Bromide Psychoses.—This is very simple. The drug itself is withdrawn, and instead table salt is given in 15 grain doses four times a day, the chloride ion thereby replacing the bromide radical in the tissues. Ample fluids and saline cathartics are added, and chloral hydrate 15 grains, is useful in promoting rest and sleep. The symptoms usually disappear within three weeks. The adrenal cortical hormone may be given in severe bromide intoxication because it appears to hasten the replacement of the bromide by the chloride radical in the tissues.

Barbituric Acid Intoxication

There are on the market many preparations of this drug, of which barbital and veronal are most frequently employed. Most of them tend to accumulate slowly in the tissues, particularly when taken for the relief of emotional tension or insomnia or when administered to control a noisy, psychotic patient. These drugs are frequently taken in enormous single doses by unstable people with the intent of committing suicide.

Early stages of intoxication are announced by a muscular incoordination with ataxia, dizziness, nystagmus, a slurred speech, and a silly, sluggish mentality. The patient acquires many bruises by falling or stumbling against walls and furniture. In more profound barbituric acid intoxication, there are varying degrees of stupor, speech is incoherent, memory is defective, and hallucinations may appear. When aroused, the patient is usually very irritable, ugly, resistive, manifesting a psychosis of a delirious type. Recovery may be very slow and may leave in its wake a mild degree of permanent dementia.

Treatment of Barbital Intoxication.—Treatment consists of withdrawal of the drug. In acute intoxication small doses of strychnine by hypodermic may have some value. Prolonged bed rest, saline catharsis, and a high caloric diet are the best restorative measures.

Intoxication With Marihuana

The use of this easily obtained drug, related to *Cannabis indica,* has aroused considerable concern in recent years. It is usually absorbed by smoking in the form of cigarettes called "reefers." After inhalation it causes a state of exhilaration and euphoria. Under its influence the victim feels light in body as if he were floating freely through space, and the general behavior is not unlike a mild mania. Instincts are freed of inhibition and sexual assaults are the most common crimes of violence attributed to the drug. The effect is short-lived, but in individuals of a psychopathic temperament there may develop a chronic dementia. Psychoses due to atropine, hyoscine, belladonna, and *Cannabis indica* infrequently occur and generally resemble the effects of marihuana.

Reference

Strecker and Ebaugh: Clinical Psychiatry, ed. 4, Philadelphia, 1935, P. Blakiston's Son & Co., Inc.

Questions for Chapter XV
Delirious Reaction Types—Drug Psychoses

1. What drugs are taken most commonly in sufficient quantities to produce drug intoxications?
2. Describe the outstanding personality defects of the chronic morphine addict.
3. Describe the "withdrawal symptoms" in morphine addiction.
4. What can the nurse do to alleviate these withdrawal symptoms?
5. How is morphine addiction treated?
6. Why are bromide and barbituric acid intoxications so common?
7. What are the symptoms of overdosage of bromides?
8. How many barbituric acid preparations can you name?
9. What are the symptoms and treatment of barbital intoxication?
10. What may be the effect of marihuana on a person of psychopathic temperament?

CHAPTER XVI

ORGANIC REACTION TYPES—PSYCHOSES WITH SYPHILIS OF THE CENTRAL NERVOUS SYSTEM

Syphilis of the nervous system in any form is due to an invasion by the organism known as *Treponema pallidum*. As it enters the brain by way of the blood, the reactions to its toxic effects vary in the different tissues it encounters, and this gives rise to different clinical diseases. Syphilis of the nervous system is roughly divided into (1) predominantly meningeal types, (2) predominantly vascular types, and (3) predominantly encephalitic types.

Meningeal Type of Syphilis

This form of syphilitic disease occurs about two or three years after the primary sore. There is a thickening of the meninges, particularly about the base of the brain. This low grade inflammation frequently injures the cranial nerves as they pass through the brain coverings, particularly the optic, oculomotor, and facial nerves. The most frequent symptoms are persistent headache, dizziness, blurring or doubling of vision, ptosis of one lid, and facial weakness. Mental symptoms such as lethargy, confusion, and stupor develop only if the pressure within the cranium becomes greatly increased. The spinal fluid always shows an increased cell count.

All these disturbances rapidly fade after a few injections of arsphenamine. To prevent more serious complications, a prolonged and intensive antisyphilitic treatment is absolutely necessary.

Vascular Type of Syphilis

Within five years after the initial infection, particularly in the absence of early and vigorous treatment, a syphilitic patient may show symptoms which indicate a disease of the cerebral arteries. The larger vessels are usually involved in the form of inflammation of the walls, narrowing of the lumen, and destruction of the inner lining. Thrombosis is the immediate accident leading to softening and degeneration of that portion of the brain tissues which depends upon the particular artery for its blood supply.

Nocturnal headaches, insomnia, and dizziness are warning signs. Over a period of several hours or days, the patient finds himself developing a hemiplegia. A slowly developing "stroke" in a younger adult is almost invariably syphilitic in origin. Loss of consciousness is not common, but speech defects are frequently associated with the hemiplegia, particularly if the paralysis is on the right side. The spinal fluid shows an increased protein content, and in most instances there is a positive Wassermann reaction.

Treatment with bismuth, arsphenamine, and iodides usually leads to a definite improvement in both mental and physical signs unless the damage to the brain has been too extensive. Again it cannot be overemphasized that continued therapy for a long period is necessary to prevent recurrences or to avoid deeper involvement of the brain tissues.

Encephalitic Type (General Paresis)

General paresis is variously known as dementia paralytica, general paralysis of the insane, or syphilitic meningo-encephalitis. It is a progressive syphilitic infiltration of the brain tissues leading to a degeneration of nerve elements and producing typical neurological and mental disturbances.

General paresis develops within two to twenty years after the first stage of the infection. It is much more frequent in the male. About 10 per cent of all admissions to a mental hospital are for general paresis.

The early signs of this disease are so insidious in appearance that they may be unrecognized even by intimate friends until an acute episode of some sort occurs. This may be a convulsion, or the full-blown symptoms may appear only after severe injury to the head.

Gradual changes in personality are the principal features of the very early phase. The patient becomes forgetful in keeping appointments, is careless of his dress, shows a general coarseness in the finer social graces. Judgment becomes poor, and there is a tendency to evade important issues, to show a smug indifference or apathy to critical problems. General mental deficiency is covered by shallow rationalizations, by outbursts of irritability, and by moods of depression or elation.

In the complete mental picture of general paresis, the outstanding feature is a feeling of grandeur. Delusions of wealth or power and euphoric ideas about the future are freely expressed. The patient plans enormous projects involving millions of dollars. He promises to build hospitals of solid gold, enormous airplanes which will cross the continent in five minutes, etc. He seems utterly unable to realize the ludicrous nature of his claims. A few patients may be depressed rather than elated. Memory defects are prominent; irritability is easily invoked when attempts are made to control the expansive ideas; and the mood is unstable.

Physically the signs are equally typical. The pupils are irregular; there is a marked tremor of the lips and.

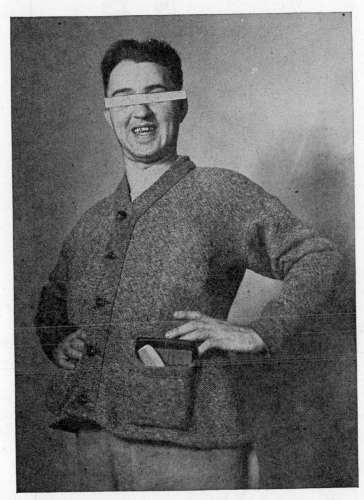

Fig. 24.—A patient with general paresis showing an exalted, silly mood.

Tabes Dorsalis or Locomotor ataxia —
Occurs five to fifteen yrs. after infection
clumsiness of feet & legs. Tendency to stagger when
in dark — Severe cramping pains in limbs —
(stabbing)
stabbing pains in abdomen about same time —
called Gastric crisis. Pains subside in course
of several years — Gradually gait becomes unsteady
Legs numb & weak — Vision may fail them —
Inability to control bladder — If not treated becomes
invalid —

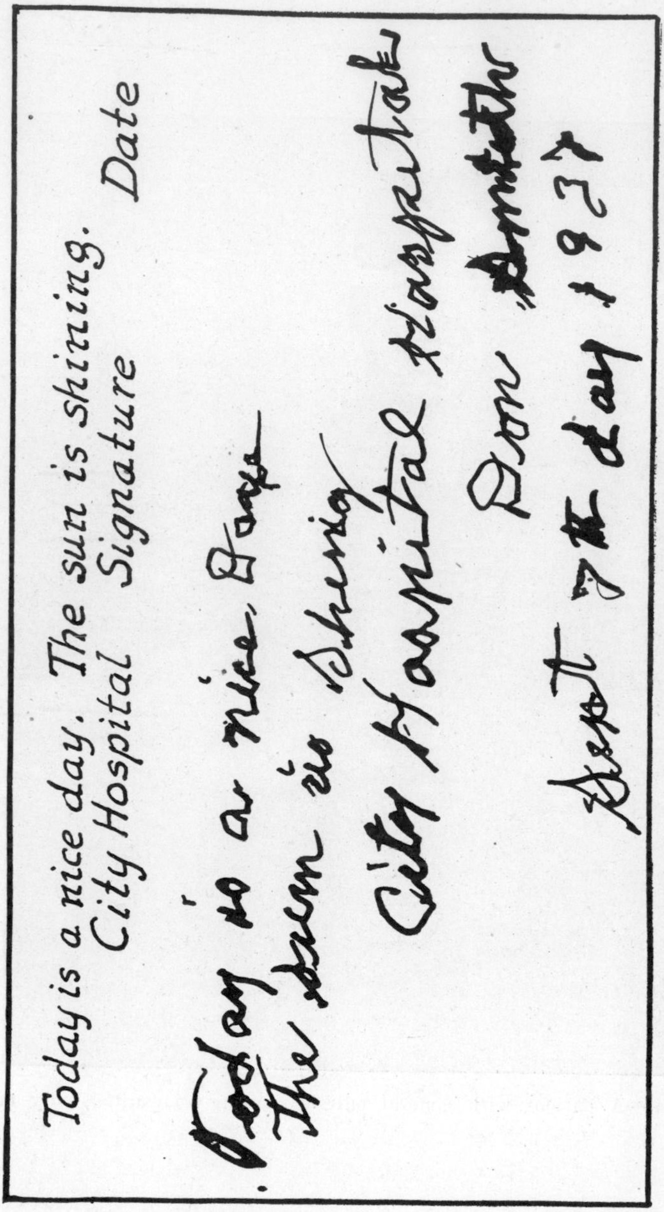

Today is a nice day. The sun is shining.
City Hospital   Signature   Date

Today is a nice day.
The sun is shining.
City Hospital Hospital
Don Smith
Sept 7th day 1937

Fig. 25.—Sample of writing in general paresis.

Flabby appearance to entire body.

tongue. The speech function is badly disturbed, for words are slurred, syllables or even words are omitted, and certain phrases are unpronounceable. Writing is likewise disturbed. Incontinence of urine and absence of the tendon reflexes generally indicate that the process has involved the cord in the form of tabes dorsalis.

The laboratory tests are most valuable in confirming the diagnosis. In the greater majority of cases the blood shows a positive Wassermann reaction. The critical test lies in an examination of the spinal fluid which is almost universally Wassermann positive; the cell count varies

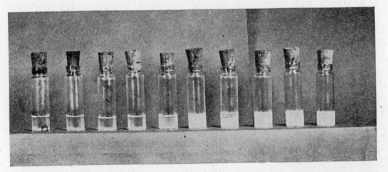

Fig. 26.—The colloidal test of the spinal fluid in general paresis. The test was performed with gum mastic and the first four tubes show a complete precipitation. These are read as 5; the fifth tube shows only a moderate degree of precipitation and is read as 3; the last five tubes are normally milky or opalescent and the reading in each is zero. Hence the total reading is 5555300000.

from 10 to 200 cells per cubic centimeter and the globulin content is greatly increased. The so-called colloidal test performed either with gold chloride or gum mastic reveals the paretic curve which is recorded generally as 5555542100.

Unless the patient with general paresis is drastically treated, the outcome is a progressive degeneration of mind and body so that he leads the existence of a vegetable, requiring the care necessary for a helpless child.

Death occurs within six to eight years after the mental symptoms set in.

The main symptoms outlined above may be associated with a great variety of other manifestations. A fairly typical demonstration of general paresis is afforded in the following story:

J. P., aged 48 years, was a building contractor who had a fairly successful business, owned his home, and had three normal children. Up to six months before admission he had been a dutiful husband and father and had a good reputation for veracity and honesty. He first manifested a change in personality when he insisted that he knew more about house plans than his architect and proceeded to draw up sketches which were obviously full of errors. He made promises to furnish apartments for owners which he could not possibly keep. He used coarse language in the presence of his children and was careless about his wearing apparel. He drove his car recklessly and finally wrecked it against a concrete trolley pole. The week before admission he purchased a huge assortment of expensive furniture which he insisted on installing in a small four-room apartment. The following day he ordered a carload of butter for his home and tried to cash a check for $30,000. He was arrested because he argued violently with the bank teller who refused him the money.

To the admitting nurse he confided that he was planning to build a thousand apartments, rent them for a dollar a month, and build a thousand more. He offered to buy solid gold instruments for the physician who examined him. He denied being sick and insisted on being permitted to call up the mayor by phone. His pupils were small and failed to react to light; the lips and facial muscles were extremely tremulous. When asked to repeat the test phrase, "The electricity in the Methodist Episcopal Church," his response was, "The elestry of the Mestiple Church." The knee and ankle reflexes were greatly exaggerated. His writing was scarcely legible.

The spinal fluid Wassermann was strongly positive; there were 80 cells, and the colloidal mastic curve was read as 5554432100.

By way of treatment he was given ten malarial paroxysms followed by 3 grams of tryparsamide weekly for eight weeks. Iodide of potassium in 10 minim doses three times a day was also administered. Within two months after admission his conduct was vastly improved. He was no longer grandiose and had gained considerable insight; there was a moderate improvement in speech and writing ability. He was discharged to his wife as moderately improved.

Treatment of General Paresis.—Nothing has proved so effective in retarding this serious brain disease as the application of some fever-producing agent. The inoculation of tertian malaria, a treatment developed by Wag-

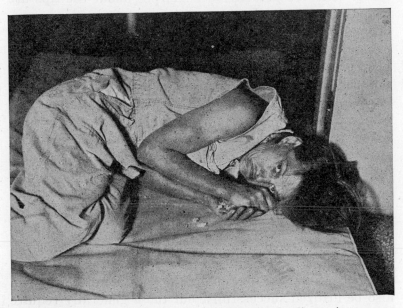

Fig. 27.—General paresis. An advanced form of the disease in a woman who is untidy, vulgar and mentally deteriorated.

ner-Jauregg in 1917, has been most enthusiastically adopted and appears to be more promising than any other so far introduced. Since its inception the number of improved or arrested cases has risen from 3 or 4 per cent to nearly 33 per cent.

Five cubic centimeters of blood are taken from a patient with active malaria and inoculated into the vein, or under the skin, of the patient. After an incubation period varying from a few days to four or five weeks, the patient has a chill and a high fever which subsides within a few hours. The paroxysm recurs every other day, during which the patient should be in bed. The temperature, pulse, and respiration should be recorded every thirty minutes until the fever subsides. Frequently during the height of the fever the paretic patient becomes confused or delirious. Herpes about the lips are frequently noted. In case of extreme cyanosis, irregular pulse, and other signs of collapse, caffeine sodium benzoate, 3 grains, can be administered hypodermically. Five grains of quinine sulphate by mouth may reduce the severity of the symptoms and may repress a succeeding paroxysm. A moderate degree of jaundice may appear, and a definite anemia is almost always present. After eight or ten paroxysms are permitted, the malarial effect is terminated by oral administration of quinine sulphate, 15 grains a day, for four days, and half that amount for four additional days. Relapses of malarial fever are practically unknown after this routine.

In cases in which malaria inoculation is unavailable or there appears to be an immunity to the organism, typhoid protein shock may be substituted. Various mechanical devices for raising the body temperature can also be utilized successfully, but these generally require on the part of the patient a degree of cooperation of which he is often incapable.

After the fever therapy, all patients should have a long course of treatment with arsenical compounds. Of these, undoubtedly the most useful is tryparsamide. This is given in 2 or 3 gram doses by intravenous injection weekly for sixteen weeks. This drug should not be given in cases where atrophy of the optic nerve exists. Finally, the therapeutic program should include an alternating series of intramuscular injections of bismuth

Induction 1st stage - Humidity
Pt goes into cabinet practically nude - T. & Resp - q 15 min
Maintenance period - Complications - tetany - tingling of hands & ft.

SYPHILIS OF CENTRAL NERVOUS SYSTEM   195

Calcium glutamate for tetany

subsalicylate in oil (2 grains) and tryparsamide injections extending over several years. Not until the spinal
fluid shows a negative Wassermann reaction and its protein content is sharply reduced can one say that the
process is arrested. Even then a complete return to normal mental acuity is rarely possible.

pulse 160 - always take pt out of regardless

References

Bing, Robert: Textbook of Nervous Diseases, translated and enlarged
    by Webb Haymaker, St. Louis, 1939, The C. V. Mosby Company.
Grinker, Roy R.: Neurology, Springfield, Ill., and Baltimore, Md., 1934,
    Charles C. Thomas.
Strecker and Ebaugh: Clinical Psychiatry, ed. 4, Philadelphia, 1935,
    P. Blakiston's Son & Co., Inc.

Questions for Chapter XVI

Organic Reaction Types—Psychoses With Syphilis of the Central Nervous System

1. What is the cause of syphilis of the nervous system?
2. Distinguish between the meningeal, vascular, and encephalitic types.
3. What are the early signs of general paresis?
4. What are the later mental and physical symptoms?
5. Are all general paretic patients euphoric? Explain.
6. What are the laboratory findings if general paresis is present?
7. What type of fever-producing therapy seems to be most efficacious in treating general paresis?
8. Outline the nursing care of a patient treated with malarial therapy.
9. How are the malarial paroxysms terminated after the patient has had sufficient treatment? Give dosage.
10. What chemotherapy is usually employed in treating general paresis?
11. Is it important to continue this treatment after malaria has been terminated? Why?

Chemotherapy - Neoarsphenamine -
Erchlike? -
Fever therapy pyrotherapy - 1916 - typhoid
1. malaria
2. Typhoid
3. Fever Cabinet - 1917
4. Continuous tub -
arrests infection & inhibit growth of bacteria
increases white count.
Give NaCl₂ + Vitamin B - after fever therapy

CHAPTER XVII

ORGANIC REACTION TYPES—THE TRAUMATIC PSYCHOSES

In the present era of heavy industries and congested traffic conditions, injuries to the head have become of frequent occurrence and unfortunately leave in their wake a wide array of mental and nervous disorders which are not always easy to evaluate.

The immediate consequences of injury to the head are not of direct interest to the psychiatric nurse or the psychiatrist. The management of those who come to the hospital after trauma to the head is a problem for the surgeon and the neurologist.

However, it is of prime importance to understand the significance of acute brain injury in relation to mental changes which may immediately or remotely follow it. A severe blow on the head generally causes the condition known as *concussion*. This is a transitory or prolonged period of unconsciousness, accompanied by signs of shock. The temperature may be subnormal, the blood pressure low, the pulse feeble and irregular. The pupils are often irregular in shape, different in size, and respond poorly to light. Vomiting of a projectile type frequently occurs. In severe cases of concussion the brain is the site of many small hemorrhages.

Bleeding from a large vessel may cause a rapid rise in intracranial pressure, a rigid neck, and progressive stupor. The spinal fluid in such instances is grossly bloody. A paralysis of one or both limbs on one side generally indicates a laceration of the brain tissues.

Recovery depends on the degree of shock and upon the amount of damage to the brain and the blood vessels.

Unconsciousness or semistupor may endure for many days or even weeks before the patient becomes clearly aware of the surroundings.

Patients who recover from the immediate effects of trauma to the head show varying disturbances after a time, which become complex diagnostic problems for the reason that many different factors enter into the situation. Not only must the amount of actual damage to the brain be considered, but the type of personality involved, the social and financial situations which existed before as well as after the injury are contributing elements in the final mental picture. All these must be carefully analyzed, for a great number of these injuries become matters of controversy in court rooms and before industrial compensation boards. A number of classifications are in use; the following are the main types encountered in ordinary psychiatric practice:

True Traumatic Encephalopathy

This implies a definite brain injury resulting in progressive deterioration. There need be no actual paralysis, and generally there is no outward evidence of physical damage. However, the patient gradually shows marked personality change. Emotional instability, lack of normal interest, general indifference, outbursts of vile temper, and a disposition to slothfulness are the outstanding symptoms. Epileptic attacks are common. Memory defects can be demonstrated as well as inability to focus the attention upon any productive work. These patients gradually gravitate to institutions for treatment.

Post-Traumatic Constitution

This represents a lesser degree of direct brain injury and the exact mechanism responsible for the symptoms

is not understood. The patient complains of various
head symptoms, among which the most common are insomnia, head pains, head noises, dizziness, and inability
to concentrate. Physical signs are usually absent. This
vague disorder is unfortunately the most common after-
math of head injury, about 50 per cent belonging to this
group. In the majority of cases, these distressing symptoms gradually fade. Where, however, the situation is
complicated by litigation and desire for compensation
for injury, the affliction may become exaggerated and
prolonged by unconscious elements of an hysterical nature, making it a chronic nervous state.

Post-Traumatic Psychoneurosis or Hysteria

In this condition there may be little or no basis for
believing that brain damage exists. It is essentially a
defense mechanism by which the patient unconsciously
develops physical symptoms after a slight head injury
to gain security against poverty, to obtain more agreeable occupation, or to be adequately compensated for
what he believes to be a grievous injury. The symptoms
are generally brought into being by the suggestion of
well-meaning friends and relatives. The average, poorly
informed individual has many dreadful ideas about the
brain and its sensitivity to damage; his fears that something dire may happen make him apprehensive and pan-
icky; and such panic is readily converted into bizarre
physical symptoms which have only a vague relation
to the injury. Frequently old anxieties and problems
are also converted into physical troubles and are assigned to the alleged injury. The patient is not a true
malingerer, for to him his symptoms are genuine. He
is rarely conscious of the fact that such symptoms are
evolved out of his desire to escape from his general in-

security about his social and financial problems, although at times he may consciously enlarge upon his so-called physical defects and be overly anxious to demonstrate them. Here the recovery occurs only as rapidly as his sense of panic and uncertainty about income, social status, and personal matters can be assuaged.

Treatment and Nursing Care.—The treatment of a psychosis which follows severe brain damage and which results in gradual deterioration is largely one of the routine custodial type. Bromides and barbital preparations in average doses are recommended for those periods when the patient manifests a mood of irritability and excitement, but these should be dispensed with as soon as such episodes subside. It is better that such patients occupy quiet quarters away from relatives and other patients to prevent outbursts of petulance and paranoid reactions. Emotional demonstrations of any sort should be avoided as much as possible. Some simple form of occupation which makes little demand for sustained physical or mental effort does much to keep the patient contented and free from wide mood swings. If convulsions occur at frequent intervals, it is necessary to administer phenobarbital continuously in appropriate doses, averaging 2 grains a day.

The treatment and the management of those patients with the so-called traumatic constitution vary only in minor details from that which applies to those who have had unquestionable brain injury. Sedatives should not be freely given, for the patient is prone to habit formation. More important is a restful environment free from noise, for noise is badly tolerated and aggrevates the head symptoms. Assurance that such symptoms are not indicative of dire disorder within the head is of greatest psychological value. Strenuous physical exercise involving quick movements of the head or excessive emotional tension should be likewise avoided. Tepid baths at night and cold wet packs to the head offer much symptomatic relief.

Quite different is the nursing care of those who have the hysterical symptoms as a consequence of head injury. Treating each individual symptom should be tactfully avoided, for a maneuver of this sort will strengthen the patient's conviction that he is physically ill. Moreover, the nurse must be careful in her manner and speech so that nothing which is said or done can be construed by the patient as further evidence that his symptoms are grounded on true injury. The hysteric patient wants sympathy, much attention and seeks confirmation from authority that he is very ill. It is of prime importance to lead the attention of the patient from his subjective miseries to outside interests. At the same time the nurse should not assume a brusque or scornful attitude carrying the idea that the patient is feigning his troubles. Simple recreations such as games, the less strenuous athletic contests, and walking are admirable methods of helping the hysteric patient to develop self-confidence and to carry his interests away from his nervous symptoms. Only strictly indicated medication should be given.

Reference

Brock, Samuel: Injuries of the Skull, Brain and Spinal Cord, Baltimore, 1940, Williams & Wilkins Company.

Fetterman, Joseph L.: The Mind of the Injured Man, Chicago, 1943, Industrial Medicine Book Co.

Gross, Sidney W., and Ehrlich, Wm.: Diagnosis and Treatment of Head Injuries, New York, 1940, Paul B. Hoeber, Inc.

Monro, Donald: Cranio-Cerebral Injuries, New York, 1938, Oxford University Press.

Rowbotham, G. F.: Acute Injuries of the Head, Baltimore, 1942, Williams and Wilkins Co.

Questions for Chapter XVII

Organic Reaction Types—The Traumatic Psychoses

1. What are the symptoms of brain concussion?
2. Discuss true traumatic encephalopathy.
3. What are the symptoms in post-traumatic constitution?
4. Give the important features in post-traumatic hysteria.
5. Which of the three types of traumatic psychoses is most common?
6. What is a malingerer? Is the patient with post-traumatic hysteria malingering?
7. What is the difference in nursing care of a patient with a real traumatic psychosis and one with the hysterical type?
8. Why should sedatives be avoided?
9. What are some methods by which the nurse can turn her patient's interests from himself to outside activities?

CHAPTER XVIII

ORGANIC REACTION TYPES—PSYCHOSES WITH BRAIN TUMOR AND OTHER BRAIN DISEASES

A number of common brain diseases are recognized by a combination of mental and neurological signs. In these the mental features are as important from the diagnostic and therapeutic standpoint as are the other symptoms.

Psychoses With Brain Tumor

The mental features of brain tumor are extremely varied and are largely determined by the site, the nature, and the size of the growth. However, when the tumor is large enough to increase greatly the pressure within the skull, irrespective of its nature or position, the symptoms are generally those of mental sluggishness, poor attention, irritability, and a tendency to lethargy and stupor. Such symptoms are usually associated with headache, choked discs, and vomiting of a projectile type. These three signs are quite constant features of brain tumor.

In tumors of the frontal lobe the patient usually shows marked personality changes: he becomes silly, unstable emotionally, and inclined to shallow facetiousness or jocosity, a condition called *Witzelsucht*. Frequently another outstanding symptom may be a grand mal form of epilepsy.

Tumors of the temporal region may produce a number of interesting mental signs, but these are commonly associated with peculiar sensory symptoms. These pa-

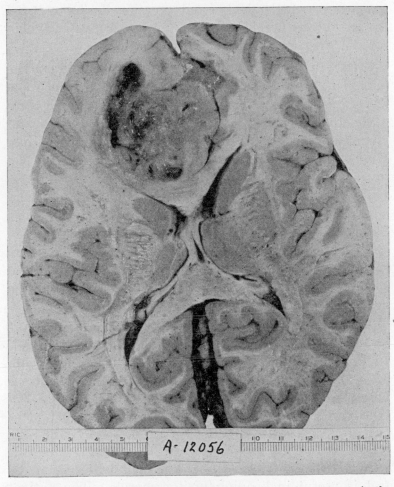

Fig. 28.—Horizontal section of the brain, demonstrating a tumor in the frontal region. This is a glioma which invades the white matter, causing personality changes, convulsions, and increased intracranial pressure.

tients often complain of attacks of epilepsy announced by queer sensations of smell, by flashes of light seen only to one side of the body, and occasionally by unusual dream states wherein events occur which seem vaguely familiar or seem to have happened before.

Treatment and Nursing Care of Brain Tumors.—The patient with brain tumor should be kept in a quiet room and should be spared from all sudden jarring or physical commotion as much as possible. The headache and stupor can be controlled frequently by keeping the patient quiet and applying a cold wet pack or an ice bag to the head. Hypertonic sugar solution given intravenously aids in reducing the intracranial pressure and is particularly recommended as a postoperative routine. Saline cathartics to keep the bowel content watery are also useful. Water intake should be reduced to no more than 1000 c.c. to control further the headache and mental confusion. Sedatives should be given with great caution because these may conceal important diagnostic signs.

The above routine applies as well to patients who have had an operation for brain tumor. In addition, hypnotics can be administered to prevent undesirable excitement and excessive movement. The dressings about the head must be protected from manipulation by the patient. In the convalescent period, the patient should be encouraged to sit up, and, if vision is not badly impaired, simple diversions such as sewing and weaving are advisable. Reading aloud to the patient with visual defect is useful in keeping up the morale. The patient recovering from brain tumor requires a long period of slow and patient rehabilitation. Any activity demanding long and intense concentration must be avoided; there must be a wide variety of simple diversions and activities.

Psychosis With Multiple Sclerosis

Multiple sclerosis has become one of the most common diseases of the brain and spinal cord within the last three decades. The condition may come on abruptly or gradually and disables its victims by causing a spastic paralysis of the lower extremities, a marked tremor of the hands, and a nystagmus. Mental changes occur in the advanced and chronic forms. These consist largely of great emotional instability, a tendency to euphoria or a false mood of gaiety, and a general unconcern about the gravity of the physical symptoms. This may be accompanied by gradual blunting of mental acuity in general and a progressive tendency to sluggishness and indifference.

Treatment is largely symptomatic and custodial because the exact cause of this affliction is unknown. Because of the coarse tremor such patients must frequently be fed by hand. Fortunately bedsores are not common. The patient must be protected from disastrous falls, for walking is usually an awkward, swaying performance. A wheel chair is usually the most sensible vehicle for the patient with multiple sclerosis.

Psychoses With Epidemic Encephalitis

This condition is probably due to a virus infection of the brain. In the acute phase the patient is delirious and feverish and often complains of diplopia. These symptoms are usually followed by a long period of lethargy which may last for several days and in rare instances for several months. Hence the disease is often called "sleeping sickness." In children who have contracted the disease, behavior disorders are outstanding, such as wild outbursts of rage and noisy respiration. In adults the end results are usually a gradual spasticity of the limbs, a constant tremor of the hands, a masklike expression, and a drooling of saliva from the mouth— a condition known as parkinsonism. The mental disturbances are usually secondary to the patient's muscular rigidity and general physical helplessness. Irritability, moroseness, frequent bodily complaints, and insomnia are the most common features. True mental deterioration rarely occurs except in the very advanced cases.

The treatment of the parkinsonism with hyoscine does much to relieve the stiffness, fatigue, and drooling. Hyoscine hydrobromide can be given by mouth, 1/150 grain, two or three times a day. Stramonium, in 5 grain doses, three times a day has the same beneficial effect. In addition to the hyoscine or stramonium, a morning dose of $\frac{1}{6}$ grain of amphetamine sulphate should be given to induce more animation and to resist fatigue.

Sedatives are helpful for irritability and insomnia. The nursing care of the patient with the chronic form of encephalitis is largely custodial in type. Mild exercise is to be alternated with long periods of bed rest. The patient should be encouraged to feed himself even though the procedure requires an extra amount of time. The food should be solid, for because of the constant tremor the patient cannot manage soups or semisoft material. The parkinsonian patient must never be hurried, and a great deal of patience on the part of the nurse in assisting him in all necessary maneuvers will be greatly appreciated. Occupational therapy is not recommended unless the tremor is mild, and the medical treatment allows a great deal of muscular relaxation.

Psychoses With Huntington's Chorea

This is a hereditary brain disease, first described by an American physician in 1872. The symptoms usually develop in middle life with twitching of the face and with purposeless movements of the trunk and limbs. These movements become more pronounced and constant, so that in severe cases the sufferer can no longer feed or dress himself. There is frequently evidence of slow intellectual deterioration and personality changes expressed by irritability and outbursts of temper. Occasionally the patient expresses ideas of reference and delusions of persecution. Attempts at suicide are common because the patients soon become aware of the hopelessness of their condition.

There is no specific treatment for this disease. Occasionally some of the patients show symptomatic improvement with the use of scopolamine, which is given once a day in doses of 1/60 grain by mouth. Institutional care is recommended because the seclusion it affords tends to reduce the motor restlessness. Tepid baths also help in suppressing the choreic symptoms. Sedatives, such as bromides, in average doses should be given regularly if the patient is unduly noisy or resistive.

References

Bailey, Percival: Intracranial Tumors, Springfield, Ill., and Baltimore, Md., 1933, Charles C. Thomas.

Cushing, Harvey: Intracranial Tumors, Springfield, Ill., and Baltimore, Md., 1932, Charles C. Thomas.

Karinthy, Frigyes: A Journey Round My Skull, New York, 1939, Harper & Brothers.

Sachs, Ernest: The Diagnosis and Treatment of Brain Tumors, St. Louis, 1931, The C. V. Mosby Company.

Questions for Chapter XVIII

Organic Reaction Types—Psychoses With Brain Tumor and Other Brain Diseases

1. What determines the mental symptoms of brain tumor?
2. What symptoms of intracranial pressure are usually present in advanced cases of brain tumor?
3. Distinguish between the symptoms of brain tumor in the frontal lobe and that in the temporal lobe.

208   PSYCHIATRY FOR NURSES

4. What are the important points in the nursing care of a patient with brain tumor, both preoperatively and postoperatively?
5. What are the physical-mental symptoms of multiple sclerosis?
6. Should patients with multiple sclerosis be allowed to walk up and down stairs alone?
7. Discuss epidemic encephalitis as to cause, symptoms, and treatment.
8. What symptoms are characteristic of parkinsonism?
9. At what time of life do symptoms of Huntington's chorea usually develop?
10. Is the disease considered to be hereditary?
11. Why must the nurse be especially tactful in caring for patients with Huntington's chorea?

CHAPTER XIX

ORGANIC REACTION TYPES—PSYCHOSES WITH CEREBRAL ARTERIOSCLEROSIS

While senile dementia and arteriosclerotic psychosis are considered as being two separate ailments, the two conditions quite frequently exist side by side. Arteriosclerotic brain disease generally appears much earlier than does true senile deterioration, the symptoms beginning sometimes as early as the fiftieth year. Actually disease of the arteries may be found in relatively young individuals. This is particularly true of the so-called malignant hypertension, a process which involves the small vessels and arterioles. A victim of this malady may expire with failure of coronary circulation, failure of kidney function, or a massive hemorrhage in the brain long before he attains old age.

Mental Symptoms of Malignant Hypertension

The patient with chronic high blood pressure develops many subjective symptoms. He suffers with head pressure and recurring headaches, has attacks of dizziness and syncope, and complains of buzzing in the ears, flashes of light before the eyes, and blurring of vision. Above all other symptoms he is subject to a great and painful anxiety, is prone to crying spells, outbursts of irritability, and an excessive preoccupation with his symptoms. Actual mental deterioration is slow to appear unless an attack of apoplexy intervenes. For years the mental acuity of the patient may remain undisturbed, and the only departures from a normal mental state are an emotional instability and a tendency to sudden swings in mood.

This mental and nervous condition, unlike senile dementia, may fluctuate for no apparent reason. There may be long periods of freedom from almost every symptom, even though the arterial disease persists and the blood pressure continues to remain high.

However, as the condition becomes more chronic, certain features can always be demonstrated if the patient is closely observed. The patient loses initiative; it becomes difficult to arouse himself to action; his endurance is diminished; and concentration becomes very trying. Gradually, disturbances of memory for recent events can be detected, but orientation is well retained until the patient becomes bedridden. Then delirium is frequent, and eventually the patient suffers frequent attacks of apoplexy or brain hemorrhage and dies of general exhaustion or congestive pneumonia. The entire process may last a few months or may extend over two decades. Hence, it is extremely difficult to offer a reliable prognosis in arteriosclerotic brain disease with hypertension, while in simple senile dementia, life expectancy is not much more than eight or ten years.

Mental Symptoms of Simple Arteriosclerosis

This is the arteriosclerosis of the more elderly patient. The blood pressure is not very high; in fact, it may be normal. The disease involves the larger arteries of the body and the brain. Large patches or plaques of fatty and calcified material appear in the inside layers of the blood vessel, gradually closing down or narrowing the channel or lumen. In the brain this may lead to anemia and sluggish circulation.

The mental symptoms are not unlike those of true senile dementia, but they may appear rather suddenly. The patient may be seized with attacks of unconsciousness, confusion, loss of speech, and temporary paralysis of one side of the body. These symptoms may gradually disappear only to recur at irregular intervals. In the meantime, general mental efficiency becomes lessened; speech shows some defects in articulation; and irritability increases. Finally, an attack of unconsciousness occurs; fever develops; and, if the patient does not expire, recovery is incomplete, and a permanent hemiplegia keeps the patient bedridden for many montns. Death occurs as a direct result of exhaustion and bronchopneumonia.

The lesion in the brain is not generally a true hemorrhage in this type of cerebral arteriosclerosis. More often it is a large area of softening where the brain tissue has degenerated because of a total blocking of the artery which supplies that particular part. The process of acute softening is therefore due to a thrombosis.

Thrombosis or softening occurs more frequently at night while the patient is asleep or after a heavy meal. Hemorrhage in the brain, on the other hand, usually occurs when the patient is excited, is hard at work, or is straining at the stool.

Treatment of Cerebral Arteriosclerosis.—Because of our ignorance of the true cause of arteriosclerosis, we cannot institute much in the way of prophylaxis against this disease. Probably the most important preventive measure is to free the patients, as far as possible, from all mental and physical exertion. This alone may result in a gratifying improvement in both the mental and physical symptoms. Emotional disturbances of any kind should be carefully avoided.

Proof is lacking that any of the usually recommended diets are useful, although execessive meat diet may be injurious. The patient should not, however, be allowed to overfill the stomach with solid or liquid food. This may lead to cerebral anemia. Strenuous procedures like

Anxiety – Depression – Suspicious .have delusions
Loss of expression defective memory
unable to speak words clearly –
Don't think accurately – Attention fixed
a difficulty ..

hot or cold baths or packs should be absolutely prohib-
ited. Mild exercise in the open air, on the other hand, is
recommended.

Above all, the arteriosclerotic patient should be given
something to keep him busy, such as sedentary occupational therapy or a small amount of ordinary house work.
This goes a long way in preventing fretting and painful
introspection.

If the blood pressure is not high and there is evidence
of failing cardiac function, digitalis is decidedly useful.
Diuretics in small doses may also produce considerable
symptomatic relief. Sedatives can be given, the barbiturates being preferred. Ascorbic acid, 200 to 500 mg.,
has also been recommended for insomnia and restlessness. If the patient becomes delirious, it is wise to administer 25 c.c. of 50 per cent hypertonic glucose by vein
once or twice a day.

The Nursing Care of Hemiplegia.—Since so many
elderly people develop hemiplegia as a result of hemorrhage or thrombosis, it is not amiss to stress a few features of the treatment of this complication. In most
instances, a few weeks after a stroke, the paralyzed side
becomes spastic, the upper and lower extremities take
on certain fixed positions. The arm is held to the side
of the body and the elbow is firmly held in a flexed position with the hand assuming a claw-like appearance.
The leg is generally found in a rigidly extended position,
and frequently some voluntary control of the lower
member is retained.

In manipulating the patient, the nurse should refrain
from pulling too vigorously at the arm and from attempting to flex or abduct the leg. This causes pain and ag-
gravates the irritability of the patient. Hemiplegic patients should have the body position shifted frequently
to prevent skin injury and bed sores. Gentle manual

massage has some value in relaxing the tonic spasm and is of decided psychological benefit. The head and chest should be elevated during the day in the same manner as one deals with the asthmatic or cardiac patient. Feeding should be a slow and patient process, for many of the sufferers with hemiplegia have some impairment in swallowing.

Presenile (Alzheimer's) Dementia

This is a rare type of dementia, which resembles that of old age but which may occur as early as the forty-fifth year. The cause is unknown. The brain shows a progressive atrophy, and the arteries may also show evidence of rapid degeneration. Memory defects are prominent mental symptoms; the mental efficiency rapidly depreciates; and convulsions occur at irregular intervals. The treatment is that which is applicable to any case of cerebral arteriosclerosis and is, therefore, largely symptomatic. *Cause unknown*

Reference

Bleuler, Eugen: Textbook of Psychiatry, translated by A. A. Brill, New York, 1924, The Macmillan Co.

Questions for Chapter XIX

Organic Reaction Types—Psychoses With Cerebral Arteriosclerosis

1. What is the important difference between arteriosclerotic psychosis and senile dementia?
2. List the physical and mental symptoms of malignant hypertension.
3. Differentiate between brain hemorrhage and thrombosis.
4. Why should we be careful of the patient's emotional state in cerebral arteriosclerosis?
5. Discuss the nursing care of the hemiplegic patient.
6. What is Alzheimer's dementia?
7. What are the physical findings in the brains of patients with cerebral arteriosclerosis? with Alzheimer's dementia?

CHAPTER XX

ORGANIC REACTION TYPES—SENILE PSYCHOSES

Old age is a natural process wherein there is a gradual lessening of mental acuity, a contraction of social interests, and an abatement of physical activity. Old people are not highly adaptable to new ideas and to drastic changes in the routine of their daily lives. Old age is associated with many bodily infirmities, bones lose their dense structure, muscles become hypertonic, and the internal organs undergo a gradual atrophy. Joints are less flexible, tremor is often present, and vision may become slowly clouded by cataract formation.

The brain of old age becomes smaller; there is always some atrophy and abnormal deposits of iron are scattered through the nerve cells. Peculiar formations called senile plaques are characteristic, and arteriosclerosis is always a concomitant condition. Yet neither arterial degeneration nor atrophy necessarily means serious senile mental decay. Here again the inability to meet personal problems seems to be the crucial factor which leads to confusion and irritability in the aging person. Arguments over property, fear of poverty, unhappy situations between parents and children are psychological reasons behind many a senile agitation. Blindness, loss of hearing, a stroke of paralysis, or some painful affliction such as a carcinoma, chronic infections, and failing circulation are equally responsible as causative factors.

Types of Senile Psychoses.—No form of senile dementia can be designated as typical, because there is a wide variation in the clinical picture. It must be remembered

214

that whenever an elderly man or woman develops a senile mental disease, he or she brings into it all his or her peculiarities which have existed throughout the life of the individual and which simply become more pronounced or exaggerated.

Simple Deterioration _old age_

Simple deterioration is the most common and blandest form of senile psychosis. This is a gradual and orderly progress toward dementia, with the following outstanding symptoms: (1) loss of memory for recent events: the doings of today are hazy while minute details of events of early life are readily recalled. This is known as retrograde amnesia. (2) Lack of impressibility: important events are no longer significant as long as they do not touch directly upon the life of the patient. (3) Tendency to reminiscence: dwelling on the life and achievements of early years and a desire to recount them frequently. (4) Intolerance of change: routine must be undisturbed, otherwise there is tension and irritability. (5) Disorientation: the year is frequently forgotten, then the day of the month, but the day of the week which more directly dictates the routine of the patient's life is generally retained. (6) Restlessness: a desire to be up and about, to travel from relative to relative, frequently getting lost in transit. (7) Insomnia: a tendency to get up in the small hours of the night and to putter aimlessly about the house. (8) Failure of judgment: an aversion to taking on new responsibilities and a tendency to withdraw into apathy and indifference.

Superimposed upon this picture of simple and progressive senile dementia there occur other symptoms which justify additional classification.

The Delirious and Confused Types

The delirious and confused types of senile psychosis occasionally occur, for the aged person is very susceptible to periods of severe mental clouding. The slightest trauma or infection may precipitate a delirium. Quite frequently it is due to the slow accumulation of drugs such as bromides or barbiturates. Mild cystitis, a septic throat, bronchitis, or auricular fibrillation can be immediately responsible for acute confusion. A fractured femur is almost certain to produce it. There may be a high fever. The patient is extremely restless, recognizes no one, is combative, resistive, and incoherent. This is accompanied by complete disorientation as to time and place. This condition is generally a critical one, and the patient may expire with signs of congestive pneumonia.

The Depressed and Agitated Types

This may be nothing more than a torpid state, manifested by a desire to be left alone, to sit in dull apathy, and to avoid conversation even with relatives. Delusions in keeping with a melancholic state are common. Almost all such depressed old men and women express ideas of poverty and have a feeling that they are headed for the poor house or that they shall soon pass away. They may also become self-accusatory, with delusions of great sin. Suicidal impulsions are expressed, and morbid ideas about cancer, syphilis, and other grievous diseases are entertained. They often express the idea that they are unwanted, are "in the way," and are senseless burdens to their children.

The Paranoid Types

Some types of senile dementia are dominated by delusions of persecution and by hallucinations of smell, vision, and hearing. They are said to be latent forms of schizophrenia. The patient becomes very suspicious, turns on the relatives and accuses them of poisoning; he smells noxious gases in his room, there are prowlers about the house, etc. The behavior is further modified by periods of mutism and catatonia, the patient standing in stereotyped postures and indulging in senseless mannerisms and rituals.

The Presbyophrenic Type

Presbyophrenia is a most engaging form of senile deterioration. It occurs in people who have been lively, aggressive, jovial types in their younger days. As senility progresses, they show a peculiar excitation and become engaged in purposeless activity. They fuss incessantly, with a great show of pleasant preoccupation, carrying things from one place to another, packing their belongings together in order to "go home." They collect rubbish, attaching great significance to worthless gadgets. There is an obsessive desire to indulge in some pretended occupation, such as folding and unfolding pieces of cloth as if the patient were ironing. Bed clothes are pulled apart, folded, twisted, tied in bundles and rubbed together as if they were going through the process of washing. Together with this "occupational delirium" there is a total disorientation and gaps in recent memory are filled with patches of experiences which actually occurred twenty or thirty years before. In other words, these old people telescope their well-retained recollections into the blurred events of yesterday and today. The prognosis is generally very bad, for presbyophrenics usually exhaust themselves within one or two years.

Treatment of Senile Dementia.—Much can be done to make old age more comfortable and free of too great a degree of irritability and agitation. Precipitating factors are most important and should be given first consideration. Radical changes in living conditions, in lifelong habits of eating, resting, and working, should be avoided as much as possible. Unless the patient is very ill and infirm, old people are better off living in a detached household in their own established routine. The insistence of the younger generation that aging parents give

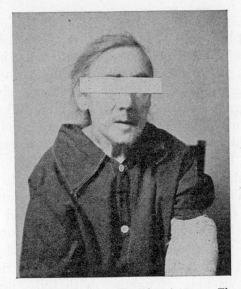

Fig. 29.—Senile dementia of the presbyophrenic type. The patient was so hyperactive that she fell and sustained a fracture of the left elbow.

up their outmoded ways of living creates constant friction and may be the prime cause of senile excitement and irritability.

To promote freedom from pain and discomfort, treatment of all infirmities, wherever possible, is of equal importance. Deficiency disease is a common feature of old age, leading to anemia, calcium deficiency and general debility. Hence a diet adequate in calcium and vitamins

B and D is indicated. Small amounts of dilute hydrochloric acid before meals may do considerable good. Failing vision should be investigated for possible glaucoma and cataract. The care of the respiratory system in old people is of prime importance, and where emphysema occurs, an effective expectorant containing such principles as potassium iodide and fluid extract of grindelia has a remarkable palliative effect. A failing circulation should be supported by a digitalis regimen.

Nursing Care of Senile Psychoses.—As to the management of a simple type of senile dementia, one can only say that it is largely a matter of simple hygiene and home nursing. Old people with a psychosis should be discouraged from using stairs and narrow corridors when walking about and certainly should not be allowed to walk the streets alone. A sudden fall may mean a fracture of the femur with its many complications, particularly fat embolus and hypostatic pneumonia. On the other hand, neither should they be entirely relegated to bed, for this may increase restlessness and irritability. To curb agitation in senile cases is one of the most difficult phases of the nursing problem. The temptation is to use bromide preparations, which are likely to accumulate and lead to drug delirium. It is better to administer barbiturates which are rapidly eliminated, such as sodium amytal in 1½ gr. doses two or three times a day. A larger dose may be necessary to avoid the "nocturnal excursions." Probably the safest soporific agent in seniles is an elixir of chloral hydrate in doses of 5 to 15 gr. at bedtime, although it is admitted that this drug does not always produce the desired effect. Large doses of vitamin C or ascorbic acid, 300 to 500 mg., are not only harmless but may actually do better than the common drugs given to induce sleep. It is needless to point out that such stimulants as alcohol, strong coffee, or tea should be avoided.

In presbyophrenic excitement, one must be careful to refrain from too much repression of the patient. These patients are generally a cheerful lot who can be easily humored and handled with tactful understanding. It is best to allow them to engage in the more harmless activities, but it requires quick thinking and artful maneuvering to keep them from wandering about where they may meet with harm.

Frequent bathing is contraindicated for more than one reason in old age. The skin is delicate and atrophied and is easily injured by rubbing. Moreover, frequent contact with water may aggravate the dryness and tendency to scale, with the result that itching and ichthyosis become added irritations to the mental confusion and excitement.

Reference

Henderson and Gillespie: A Text-Book of Psychiatry for Students and Practitioners, London and New York, 1927, Oxford University Press.

Questions for Chapter XX

Organic Reaction Types—Senile Psychoses

1. Upon what will the picture of senile psychosis depend in various individuals?
2. What is the most common form of senile psychosis? Give symptoms.
3. What type would you watch for in an elderly patient with an acute infection?
4. What is the emotional state in the depressed and agitated type? In the paranoid type?
5. Describe a patient with the presbyophrenic type of senile dementia.
6. Explain "occupational delirium," "telescoping of memory."
7. What are some precipitating factors which might aggravate senile dementia? How would you avoid them?
8. In what way could "short memory" and "love of reminiscence" help you to care for a patient with senile dementia?

CHAPTER XXI

EPILEPSY AND PSYCHOSES WITH EPILEPSY

Epilepsy, which is simply the greek word for "seizure," is not a disease in itself, but a symptom. It is an outward manifestation of disordered brain function which is now recognized as a disturbance in the so-called brain rhythm. This cerebral dysrhythmia can be detected by the electroencephalograph, an instrument described in another chapter. The convulsion or fit is an explosive phenomenon, accompanied by a violent disturbance in the brain rhythm, by varying degrees of unconsciousness, and by a sudden discharge of motor excitement.

Injury to the brain, infection, alcoholism, and brain tumor often lead to epileptic attacks, but so far the most common form of this condition, known as *idiopathic epilepsy,* appears to be accompanied by no clearly demonstrable defect of the brain. The only positive finding which can be objectively demonstrated in the vast majority of epileptic individuals is the brain wave irregularity. Fig. 30 demonstrates the contrasting appearances of a normal brain rhythm and the slow and irregular rhythm of a minor epilepsy.

Epilepsy was known to antiquity; the Greek physicians described it accurately; and in the Middle Ages it was as common as it is today. Authorities estimate that in the United States there are over a half-million individuals who suffer with periodic convulsions, many of whom have only occasional seizures and are able to conceal the fact from even their closest friends.

The earlier epilepsy appears, the more severe and devastating are the attacks, for the condition may be

221

associated with, or lead to, mental deficiency. Convulsions which appear for the first time about the age of puberty are less likely to be complicated with serious psychic disturbances.

The *grand mal* seizure is the major epileptic attack which is so dramatic and terrifying to the onlooker. The onset is usually announced by a familiar warning or aura. This consists of a momentary dizziness, a queer feeling in the region of the stomach, or such sensory experiences as tingling in the extremities or flashes of light.

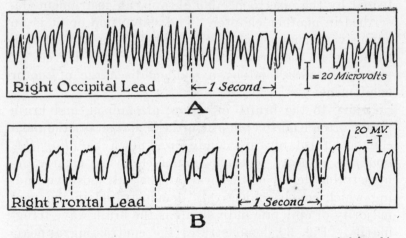

Fig. 30.—Examples of a normal and an abnormal electroencephalographic record. *A* shows normal alpha waves at the rate of 10 to 11 per second. In contrast, *B* shows large, slow waves, the so-called spike and wave discharge of 3 per second which is characteristic of a form of epilepsy.

Frequently there is a sharp gasping noise or outcry. The patient then falls suddenly and becomes completely unconscious. Serious injury may result from the fall, as every epileptic person knows from the number of scars he bears as a result of previous mishaps. As he falls, the body and limbs become rigid; the chest is fixed by this muscle spasm; respiration ceases; and the face becomes engorged and cyanotic. The pupils are widely dilated. This so-called *tonic phase* endures for 10 to 15 seconds. Urinary incontinence may occur at this time. The patient gradually relaxes and takes a deep breath, and there follows a rhythmic contraction of the muscles, a condition known as the *clonic phase*. The tongue is frequently bitten by the clamping of the jaws; the saliva accumulates in the throat and mouth and is mixed with air so that the patient "foams at the mouth." The violent contractions gradually decrease in frequency and severity. This is followed by irregular struggling gestures, fumbling of the hands, and chewing movements of the lips. A deep heavy sleep or coma ensues, which frequently lasts several hours. The patient awakes and for a time seems confused and disoriented. Headache is the chief complaint on arising, and the muscles may be painful to pressure or manipulation.

The *petit mal* is a minor attack of epilepsy. Falls are infrequent because the patient has only a momentary loss of consciousness. The attack is usually manifested by a sudden pallor of the face, a staring expression, and a short pause in conversation or movement, after which the patient resumes his normal behavior.

Jacksonian epilepsy is of interest to the neurologist because it generally means a focus of irritation in some portion of the cerebral cortex. This is an epileptic attack which involves a limited group of muscles, as the facial muscles on one side, or the facial muscles and the muscles of the upper extremity of the same side, or even the entire one side of the body. The head and the eyes are turned to the affected side; the arm and leg may be distorted by a clonic spasm. On the same side of the body the patient frequently senses peculiar tingling or crawling experiences. Consciousness is usually not lost.

Brain Pathology

For a short period after the clonic attack there may be a temporary weakness of the face, arm, or leg which was involved in the seizure.

Epileptic Clouded States

Many forms of mental upset are associated with the convulsive seizure, appearing most frequently after, but occasionally occurring before, or entirely replacing the epileptic episode. They are all regarded as varieties of epilepsy. Most common are the dreamlike or dazed states during which the patient automatically carries on complicated activities, such as driving a car through traffic or performing some technical maneuver incidental to his work. For example, a watchman may make his rounds, accurately ring all his clocks and later will recall nothing of his activity. More tragic is the epileptic furor, a sudden attack of confusion, terror, and hallucinosis during which the patient is violent, brutal, and homicidal. The sudden onset and the complete failure to recall the episode after normal consciousness returns testifies to the fact that the attack is an abnormal mental state during which the individual is not responsible for his acts.

Epileptic Dementia

In longstanding cases of epilepsy there is always some degree of intellectual blunting, although this may not be evident on superficial examination. About 30 per cent of the chronic epileptics tend to become dull, irritable, selfish, and lazy. The facial expression is often empty, the speech slow, and creative capacity is practically nil. In those unfortunate individuals where epilepsy begins early in life, the dementia may be profound, the mental capacity being so low as to require the custodial care ordinarily required for an idiot.

Treatment.—The immediate management of an individual in convulsions requires above everything else a cool head on the part of the nurse or physician. The patient should be allowed to lie on his back, the clothing should be loosened at the throat, and the mouth should be kept clear of mucus and saliva. A wad of sponge rubber or a wedge of wood covered with gauze may be inserted between the teeth to prevent injury to the tongue. If opportunity permits, the tongue itself may be seized or held with the gag to the floor of the mouth to promote freer respiration. An ice pack to the forehead may have some palliative value. Restraint of any type during the attack is decidedly harmful. A hypodermic injection of 3 grains of sodium phenobarbital is useful, particularly if there has been a long succession of such seizures. Even more efficient in stopping a series of convulsions which follow one another rapidly is the intravenous injection of 7½ grains of sodium amytal.

To reduce the severity and frequency of epileptic seizures, the bromide salts have been for many years the most successful therapeutic agents. The average epileptic patient can tolerate 25 to 75 grains of triple bromide daily, this dose giving fairly good results, particularly if the intake of table salt in the diet is very low. Appearance of a bromide rash over the face, neck or chest indicates that the drug should be withdrawn and other anti-convulsants be administered.

More popular in the last two decades have been the barbituric acid principles, such as phenobarbital. The average anticonvulsive dose is 1½ grains three times a day. Epileptic patients for some reason possess a high tolerance for this drug and rarely show signs of intoxication. The mental depression which is attributed to too much medication with phenobarbital is rarely as marked as that which is noted in heavy bromide intake.

new drug @ in past 2 years

also tridione

A newer drug whose sponsors claim for it an effective anticonvulsive value, but which does not cause a great deal of mental dullness, is sodium diphenyl hydantoinate (dilantin). In a limited number of patients, the results with this treatment have been gratifying, but its ultimate value is uncertain. It is given in three doses daily, each capsule containing 1½ grains.

Dietetic attempts to control epilepsy have not met with signal success except in children, where fasting and high-fat diets occasionally result in a definite cessation of convulsions. This ketogenic diet should be continued for at least a year in order that its benefits may be accurately determined.

Just as important as treatment with drugs is the psychological and social management of the epileptic patient. Unless there is a marked deterioration, the individual should be encouraged to maintain his self-respect and his normal place in his social group. An epileptic child should be allowed to attend public schools wherever this is possible or practical. Vigorous exercise is to be encouraged, although such hazardous pastimes as swimming or driving a car should be strictly denied. To promote every effort in planning a career and to encourage special mental and vocational training are as potent therapies, if not more valuable, than stressing the use of a drug, which should be only a measure of last resort.

References

Jelliffe and White: Diseases of the Nervous System, Philadelphia, 1935, Lea and Febiger.

Lennox, Wm. G.: Science and Seizures, New York, 1941, Harper & Brothers.

Penfield, Wilder and Erickson, Theodore C.: Epilepsy and Cerebral Localization, Springfield, Ill., 1941, Charles C. Thomas.

Putnam, Tracy J.: Convulsive Seizures, Philadelphia, 1943, J. B. Lippincott Co.

Wechsler, I. S.: A Textbook of Clinical Neurology, ed. 4, Philadelphia, 1939, W. B. Saunders Co.

Questions for Chapter XXI

Epilepsy and Psychoses With Epilepsy

1. Is epilepsy a disease or a symptom?
2. What is idiopathic epilepsy?
3. Describe a grand mal seizure.
4. What is a petit mal attack?
5. Describe Jacksonian epilepsy, epileptic clouded state, epileptic dementia.
6. What is an epileptic furor? Is there any danger from a patient with an epileptic furor?
7. What are the important points to remember in caring for a patient with an epileptic seizure?
8. What medications are helpful in controlling these attacks?
9. What type of diet occasionally aids in preventing seizures in children?
10. What psychological factors are to be considered in treating epileptic patients?

Pathological findings —

Types of Epilepsy   Vertigo, nausea —

1. Idiopathic   Grand Mal — Usual type of epilepsy
                     Petite Mal —

2.

3. Psychic equivilance

Epilepticus status. One convulsion after another —

psychic Equivalance. Very confused for an hour after attack —

CHAPTER XXII

MENTAL DEFICIENCY

Mental deficiency or feeblemindedness implies a lack of normal intellectual development that has existed from birth or was acquired early in life. It is largely a defect in understanding one's environment and in utilizing such knowledge for the purpose of social adjustment and of making a living. The person with mental deficiency is limited in his capacities and total accomplishment in direct proportion to the amount of the defect.

The menace of the feebleminded is becoming more and more apparent. It is estimated that there are over one-half million individuals in this country who are socially inadequate because of mental deficiency. Less than 3 per cent of these are confined in institutions, leaving the others at large in society.

Causes of Mental Deficiency.—The causes of mental defect can be conveniently divided into those which are hereditary or existing prior to birth, into those which result in some form of injury at the time of birth and into those which occur during the growing period.

Heredity plays an important part in the production of mental deficiency, but authorities cannot agree on the exact extent. That it plays a significant role in certain families of poor stock, particularly where syphilis or alcoholism is demonstrated, cannot be denied. Moreover, it is not yet known just how much of mental deficiency can be attributed to nutritional and infectious disease in the pregnant mother.

Injuries occurring at the time of birth arise from hemorrhage into the brain as a result of the tearing of the brain coverings and the blood vessels. It is also be-

228

lieved by some that damage to the child's brain can occur from excessive or prolonged anesthesia administered to the mother during labor. Instrumental delivery may also be responsible for damage to the cranial contents, but this is probably not as common as popularly believed.

After a child is born any number of catastrophes can arrest the development of normal intellect. Such conditions as trauma to the head, acute infections of early childhood, particularly encephalitis and meningitis, can damage the growing brain by destroying a large number of nerve cells.

Measuring Intelligence.—Mental deficiency is in part a quantitative defect and as such can be measured by so-called intelligence tests. Most of these tests—and there are many—are based on the original one devised by Binet and Simon, who studied the intellectual growth of a large number of French school children. In this country these tests have been modified by Terman, and are known as the Stanford Revision. For each year of growth beginning with the second or third year, there is a set of questions which the normal child of that year can usually answer correctly. The highest age level at which an individual can pass *all* the tests is called the basal mental age of that individual. To this are added all the tests credited in the higher age levels and the combined sum is called the mental age. Thus a child who can pass all tests on the ten-year level and half the tests on the 11-year level has a mental age of 10½ years regardless of what his chronological age may be.

For a certain class of individuals, namely those with language difficulties, i.e., foreigners, the hard of hearing, the blind, pre-school children, etc., performance tests must be used. Here intelligence is measured by mechanical behavior rather than by language response. An example of this is the Army Beta test.

Outline for Binet-Simon Tests for Intelligence

Mentality of Three Years

1. Shows eyes, nose, mouth or indicates these in pictures.
2. Repeats simple sentences with six syllables such as "It is good; I want more."
3. Repeats two digits, as 5 and 2.
4. Points out familiar objects in a simple picture.
5. Gives the family name, as Brown or Jones.

Mentality of Four Years

1. Gives own sex.
2. Names simple objects such as penny, key, spoon.
3. Repeats three digits in proper order.
4. Points out the longer of two lines on a chart.

Mentality of Five Years

1. Tells which is the heavier of two cubes which look alike.
2. Draws a square after a copy. The results should be recognized as a square.
3. Repeats ten syllables. "His name is John—he is a very good boy."
4. Counts four pennies.
5. Reassembles a card which has been cut into two triangles.

Mentality of Six Years

1. Knows the difference between morning and afternoon.
2. Defines in terms of use such words as fork, table, chair, horse, mamma. Three should be satisfactory.
3. Obeys three commands given at one time.

4. Shows the right hand and the left ear on command.
5. Can distinguish the difference between a pretty and a very ugly face.

Mentality of Seven Years

1. Counts thirteen pennies.
2. Describes a picture with fair amount of detail.
3. Notes that parts of a human figure are missing such as the eyes, nose, mouth or arms. Three should be recognized.
4. Copies a diamond so that it can be recognized as such.
5. Recognizes four colors: red, green, blue, yellow.

Mentality of Eight Years

1. Gives difference between paper and cloth, fly and butterfly, wood and glass. Time allowed, two minutes and two should be answered satisfactorily.
2. Counts backward from 20 to 1 in 20 seconds with but one error allowed.
3. Names days of the week in ten seconds.
4. Counts the value of three pennies and three two-cent stamps in ten seconds.
5. Repeats five digits in order when given but once, such as 4, 7, 3, 9, 5.

Mentality of Nine Years

1. Makes correct change from 20 cents after imaginary purchase of an article costing 4 cents.
2. Defines common objects in terms better than those of simple usage, such as fork, table, chair, house, etc.
3. Names day of the week, month, day of month and year. (Allowances may be made for missing day of month by two or three days.)
4. Names months in order in 15 seconds. One error is allowed.

Mentality of Ten Years

1. Recognizes all the coins in common circulation as well as $2, $5, and $10 bills in 40 seconds.
2. Copies two simple designs from memory, after being allowed to look at them for ten seconds.
3. Repeats six digits, as 854726, 274681, 941738.
4. Tells what one should do in certain emergencies such as presented by the questions: "What would you do if you missed a train?" or "What would you do if you broke something belonging to somebody else?" (Time allowed: 20 seconds.)
   Answers questions difficult of easy comprehension such as, "What would you do if you were asked your opinion of someone whom you did not know?" "What would you do if you were delayed in going to school?" (Time allowed: 20 seconds.)
5. Use three given words in two sentences.

Mentality of Eleven Years

1. Recognizes absurdities or nonsense in three out of five statements.
2. Uses three given words in one complete sentence.
3. Says at least 60 words in three minutes.
4. Gives three words that rhyme with "day" in 1 minute.
5. Rearranges 8 scrambled words to form a statement. (Should do two out of three with one minute for each.)

Mentality of Twelve Years

1. Repeats seven digits in order when heard but once.
2. Defines abstract terms such as charity, justice, goodness. (Two should be satisfactory.)
3. Repeats with no error a sentence of 22 to 26 syllables.

4. Resists suggestion as to which line is longer.
5. Solves problem correctly after being given facts. (Two trials must be correct.)

Mentality of Fifteen Years

1. Interprets a picture where there is some emotional situation or significant action presented.
2. Gives the correct time when hands of clock are interchanged at 6:20 or 2:56. (This test is done without the subject being allowed to see the face of a clock or watch.)
3. Given a simple code, constructs a short sentence.
4. Writes the opposite to twenty words, such as "good —bad," "light—dark," etc. Must have seventeen correct.

Mentality of an Adult (16 years and over)

1. Draws design which will appear after a piece of paper has been folded twice and a notch cut into one of the folded edges.
2. Imagines and draws the new form made by joining the transposed pieces of triangles made by cutting a rectangular card diagonally.
3. Gives difference in the meaning of abstract words such as evolution and revolution, event and advent, pride and pretence, etc. (Two correct answers are necessary.)
4. Gives three differences between the president of a republic and a king.
5. Understands the central theme in a selection read aloud by the examiner.

The Intelligence Quotient.—This is an expression of the ratio between the mental and chronological ages. Thus a child of 10 years with a mental age of 12 years will have an I. Q. of 120 per cent (12 divided by 10), and a child of 12 years with a mental age of 10 years will have an I. Q. of 83 per cent (10 divided by 12).

In measuring the intelligence of an adult it is assumed that normal adult intelligence is achieved at 16 years, although there is good evidence to believe that additional growth continues up to the twenty-second or even the twenty-third year. Hence *in estimating the I. Q. for an adult the denominator should be sixteen years* (192 months). The intelligence quotient is not an absolute index of mental capacity, but it serves as a very useful guide in predicting the potentialities in mentally backward individuals.

Wechsler-Bellevue Intelligence Scale.—This is an individual mental examination, which includes ten sub tests, five of which are verbal and five nonverbal. There are established norms for ages from 7 to 70. In addition to giving a valid measurement of intellectual capacity, it reveals significant discrepancies between performance and verbal test scores which often furnish a clew as to the quality of a psychosis. Not infrequently many important personality traits can be observed during the test interview.

The Cornell-Coxe Performance Test.—Being a nonverbal test, this can be used in cases with speech or language difficulty. It purports to measure practical reasoning and visual motor coordination.

The Minnesota Pre-school Scale.—This test can be used to measure the mental ability of children from 18 months to 6 years of age. It samples a wide range of functions, both verbal and nonverbal. It is particularly valuable in differentiating between the specific kinds of ability shown by a child. One examination yields three scores: a verbal score, a nonverbal score and a combined rating.

Types of Mental Deficiency.—The simplest classification is that based on the maximum mental development which is possible in each given case.

The *idiot* is one whose mental capacity is below the third-year level. Such children may learn to walk but are never capable of taking care of their persons in a cleanly way. They are clumsy, awkward, untidy, and require constant supervision in the performance of the simplest requirements of living. Most idiots learn a few simple words but rarely learn to talk intelligently. Various physical deformities are evident early in infancy and many of these individuals are subject to epilepsy. A certain proportion have small, cone-shaped skulls; they are known as *microcephalic idiots*.

The *imbecile* may attain a mental level of six or seven years. Imbeciles can generally talk with a very crude vocabulary, can be taught simple manual tasks, can keep themselves clean, and can protect themselves in a limited way. An imbecile cannot become self-supporting but may become useful in performing little routine chores about the home.

The *moron* ranges in mental accomplishment between the eighth-year level and the lower adult normal which is ordinarily reached at about the fifteenth year. The glaring deficiency is not so much in the ordinary mental performances but in the field of reason and judgment. Constituting more than 80 per cent of all forms of mental defect, the morons are one of the serious problems of modern times. Having no gross physical defects, they present themselves as a shiftless, unstable group which gravitates to the lowest level of manual labor and social activity. Out of this class are recruited the petty criminal, the prostitute, and the ne'er-do-well. Approximately 20 to 30 per cent of all offenders against society who are found in penal institutions belong to this borderline class of feeblemindedness.

A few special forms of mental deficiency must be included which have certain physical stigmata making them a unique clinical picture.

Amaurotic family idiocy, which occurs mainly in the Jewish race, is an idiocy accompanied by spasticity of the limbs and blindness. The symptoms generally begin about the fifth month of life and progress rapidly, the child dying within two or three years. The disease can be recognized by detecting the typical cherry-red spot in the retina of the eye. The actual cause is unknown.

Mongolian idiocy is a fairly common condition which can be recognized in the third month. The face has a mongolian cast, that is, the eyes appear to be slitlike, the face is flattened, and the skull is rounded. The tongue is enlarged and usually hangs out of the mouth, the hair is scanty, and the muscles are flabby. The fifth finger is often curved in flexion, in the so-called comma finger. The mongolian child is usually cheerful, is fond of imitating his elders, but his mental development rarely exceeds the six-year level.

The *cretin* is congenitally deficient because of inadequate thyroid secretion. Mentality is dull, and bodily growth is stunted. If treatment is instituted early enough, many of these defects can be corrected with thyroid extract.

Hydrocephalic idiots are children who develop huge heads, progressive paralysis, and mental retardation. The condition is due to obstruction of the spinal fluid pathways at the base of the brain.

Cerebral Birth Palsy.—As a result of injury at the time of birth or as a result of toxic pregnancy, the child frequently shows a spastic paralysis of the lower extremities and, with this, a mental deficiency. This condition is frequently called *Little's disease.* Coarse tremors, hemiplegia, and a condition resembling chorea may also occur in these paralytic types of feeblemindedness.

Treatment of Mental Deficiency.—It goes without saying that the very low grades of mental deficiency are institutional problems. Rarely can one entertain a hope of complete recovery. The obvious treatment is to train the retarded child to the maximum level of accomplishment. Vocational training in special schools offers the best prospects for those who have an intermediate intellectual capacity. It is doubtful whether a good environment and the best of training actually raise the intellectual quotient to any great extent, but such treatment does prepare the individual for some degree of self-support.

Nursing care in mental deficiency is largely a matter of close supervision. The nurse should emphasize a routine wherein the child will be taught cleanly habits so that his care will be less of a burden to his family. Assigning simple duties within the capacity of the patient may assist in curbing destructive tendencies. Insistence on regular bathing, washing, and correct dressing habits helps in making the feebleminded child more socially acceptable. Occupational therapy will increase the social capacity of those in the higher mental levels who are capable of some degree of manual dexterity.

References

Barr and Maloney: Types of Mental Defectives, Philadelphia, 1920, P. Blakiston's Son and Co.

Berry and Gordon: The Mental Defective, New York, 1931, Whittlesy House.

Brousseau, Kate: Mongolism, Revised by H. G. Brainerd, Baltimore, 1928, The Williams and Wilkins Co.

Goddard, H. H.: The Kallikak Family, New York, 1927, The Macmillan Co.

Wechsler, David: The Measurement of Intelligence, Baltimore, 1939, Williams & Wilkins Co.

Questions for Chapter XXII

Mental Deficiency

1. Discuss the definition of mental deficiency.
2. What are some causes of feeblemindedness?
3. How is intelligence measured?
4. Give the formula for determining the intelligence quotient.
5. Is the I. Q. an absolute index of intellectual capacity?
6. Name the three types of mental deficiency, giving the mental age level which they may attain and discuss the social adaptability of each type.
7. Explain amaurotic family idiocy, Mongolian idiocy, cretinism, hydrocephalic idiocy, cerebral birth palsy.
8. Why are close supervision and teaching advised in nursing mentally deficient patients?
9. Would you praise a feebleminded child for performing his task well?

$$\text{"I.Q."} = \frac{100 \times \text{mental age in mo.}}{\text{Chronological Age in mo.}}$$

I. Q. greater than 140 "near genius"

I. Q. - 120 - 140 = Very superior intelligence

I. Q. - 110 - 120 = Superior Intelligence -

I. Q. - 90 - 110 = Average intelligence

I. Q. 80 - 90 - Dull

I. Q. 70 - 80 - Borderline deficiency

I. Q. - Less than 70 - Feeblemindedness

I. Q. - 50 - 70 - Morons

I. Q. - 25 - 50 - Imbeciles

I. Q. - 0 - 25 - Idiots -

CHAPTER XXIII

PSYCHOPATHIC PERSONALITY

The individual with psychopathic personality is a hapless creature who on the surface appears to be normal but who seems utterly incapable of making a satisfactory social adjustment. It is a condition either hereditary, congenital, or acquired, affecting the emotional and volitional rather than the intellectual fields. The most glaring defects are a marked emotional instability, pronounced selfishness, poor judgment and insight, together with a tendency to rash and impulsive behavior.

The condition may manifest itself by a wide range of undesirable traits such as perversions in moral and sexual fields and is known by many other names such as moral imbecile, discordant personality, defective delinquent, or any term which designates the outstanding weakness in behavior, as pathological liar, kleptomaniac, pyromaniac and misanthrope.

The mental capacity in these individuals may be dull, normal, or even superior in some respects. Occasionally there is a special gift in some direction, such as music or painting.

While the patient is usually alert and even superficially brilliant, a closer study usually reveals a certain shallowness of thinking. There is a definite defect in abstract deduction, an inability to express sound views, to display calm deliberation and to think out a critical analysis of any situation. Reasoning is hasty and emotionally overloaded with ego demands. The psychopathic personality is childlike in his vivid imagery, his gullibility, and his simple-minded attempts to achieve distinction without applying himself with persistence and industry. He is notoriously incapable of sticking to his job, and changes from one occupation to another at frequent intervals.

Even in adolescence the emotional defect begins to show itself in poor application to school work; the child flies into frequent temper tantrums, is easily irritated by playmates, and suffers from violent swings in mood. There is a great desire for attention and praise, and, when this is not forthcoming, the young person feels abused and misunderstood. Total accomplishment in school or at work is poor because of lack of ambition and stability.

Antisocial behavior is the rule and consists of every form of petty misdemeanor. The behavior patterns are undoubtedly reactions to a sense of inadequacy which is only vaguely appreciated and never openly acknowledged. Because the psychopathic personality is highly egotistic, he will concede few or none of his defects and usually defends himself with ready explanations or with a defiant and sulky attitude.

Like a hunchback who feels more at ease amongst the hunchbacks, so the psychopath seeks his own kind, assumes an attitude of flippancy, and associates with a group of easier standards. Hence he becomes a rounder, a ne'er-do-well, who soon finds himself in bad company and involved in petty crime. Some maintain self-esteem through constant depreciation of others, they become world-haters, critical of everything that is good and socially correct. The sense of inferiority is translated into ideas of persecution. ''I am hounded and misunderstood, I never get a break'' is a frequent interpretation of their difficulties. There may be an overcompensation, an exaggeration of self-importance. The psychopath then brags of great achievements, Daydreaming and taking refuge in phantasy are frequently another favorite reaction because the psychopathic personality is generally blessed with a vivid and colorful imagination. The patient may become an accomplished liar, lying for the sheer joy of lying, because in the creating of his phantasies he invariably pictures himself as capable, popular, romantic and successful—everything he is not in reality. This propensity to pathological lying may develop at a very tender age. The phantasies are not true delusions, for the patient knows he is lying.

Pathological lying leads to swindling. Passing worthless checks, signing notes which will never be paid, living at expensive resorts with no concern as to costs and buying an elaborate wardrobe on credit are examples of behavior which manifest a determination to make wishful phantasy a reality.

When called to account for their irregular behavior, psychopathic personalities may show indifference, retaliate with flimsy rationalizations, or display various reactions of an hysterical nature. A common maneuver is to resort to self-pity and anxiety and to escape from responsibility by retreat into pretended illness. Often the response is an emotional explosion and a threat of suicide which is rarely carried out. In rare instances, when sorely tried, the unstable, hysteric individual with this constitutional weakness wanders off into an amnesia, forgets his identity, and appears in some distant city as a "mystery person."

Certain sexual aberrations are sometimes regarded as belonging to this general grouping of warped personality, but such perversions are not in themselves evidence of psychopathic constitution. With all his instability and naïve ego, the psychopath is not particularly given to crimes of lust, such as rape. It is true that the girl with psychopathic leanings frequently finds herself illegitimately pregnant, but this is rather the result of her desire for glamour and romance than of great sexual passion.

The character and performance of a psychopathic personality are presented in the following story:

A. M. is a young woman of 22 who was picked up by the police in the suburb of a large city because she appeared dazed and could not give her name and address. She was admitted to the observation ward of the hospital as Jane Doe. She lay quietly in bed with a vacant expression on her face. She alleged that she did not know her identity but hinted that she vaguely recalled a large mansion near New York City. She enjoyed the attention of the house physicians and very quickly elicited their sympathy by her attitude of helplessness and the air of mystery she created by her amnesia. After much prompting she managed to recall a telephone number. The exchange was found to be one belonging in the New York telephone directory but no such number was found to exist. She then talked vaguely of having graduated from the School of Journalism at Columbia University, but could not recall the names of any of her professors.

Finally the newspapers published a photograph of the "mystery girl," and a few days later a thoroughly disgusted woman came to claim the patient as her sister. At first the patient failed to recognize the visitor, but within a few hours was able to give her own name and address and to admit that the woman in question was a "relation."

It appeared that the patient had been in a hysterical fugue. She lived in a small neighboring town, had never finished high school, to say nothing of a college, and had never visited New York City.

Since her tenth year she had been a "problem child," with a reputation for touchiness and irritability. She indulged in frequent temper tantrums, was frequently given to sulks and moods, and did very poorly in school. During her second year in high school, she manifested an unusual interest in students of the opposite sex, played truant with increasing frequency, and explained her absence with fantastic stories. Repeated punishment had little or no effect on her behavior. On one occasion she disappeared from home and school for four days and was finally discovered living in a tourist camp.

She claimed she was married to an engineer who had just left for a western state on a big construction project and would not return for a year.

After suspension from school, her sister found employment for her as a package clerk in a department store. Within two months she was discharged for stealing from a glove counter. For a time she worked for short intervals as a house maid, only to be discharged shortly because she had so little sense of responsibility. She became a habitual liar, exhausted the patience of her parents, and took to staying out at night after pilfering from her mother's purse. On one occasion she became intoxicated and was detained for three weeks in a correction home for girls.

The hysterical fugue occurred after she had passed a bad check at the very store where she had previously worked. She was recognized by the store detective as a suspicious person, but, before he could detain her, she slipped out into the street, hailed a passing motorist who conveyed her to the neighboring city. Dismayed by her peculiar, detached behavior, he left her in the suburb where she was picked up by the police.

Prognosis.—Despite frequent rebuffs, sharp criticism and repeated punishment, the individual with a psychopathic personality rarely learns from experience. The very selfsame conduct which brings bitter repercussion may be repeated over and over again. He seems to be wholly unaware of the significance of a long record of misconduct and instead entertains a naïve optimism as to his real worth. In later years the psychopath finds refuge in alcohol or drugs. An unknown percentage of these people improve in social adjustment as they grow older because instinctual drives are less powerful, or there is less feeling of insecurity.

Treatment.—The management and treatment of the psychopathic personality is at best a sketchy, haphazard one. In most states the legal statutes do not allow indefinite incarceration of such patients, and the vast majority are allowed to run the gamut of reform schools, detention homes, prison, and work farms, where they do

Fetishism — Satisfaction thru feel, sight & touch.
Exhibitionism — Satisfaction thru showing self.
Homosexual — Love of own sex —

244   PSYCHIATRY FOR NURSES

very poorly. Punishment has little or no deterrent
effect, for correction cannot be directed toward the unconscious tensions which are really responsible for the
hostile and selfish behavior.

In a few cases glandular treatment has proved beneficial if endocrine deficiency has been clearly demonstrated. Fever treatment has been known to modify the
behavior favorably. Bromides and other sedatives may
be used to advantage in preventing a burst of abnormal
and impulsive activity.

If the individual is fortunate enough to possess some
special talent, training and occupation along those lines
may assuage much of the ego tension and improve social
behavior. Adjustment to a simple, monotonous routine
is impossible because by reason of his vivid infantile
emotionality, the psychopath abhors such an existence.

References

Cleckley, Hervey: The Mask of Sanity, St. Louis, 1941, The C. V. Mosby
      Co.
Henderson, D. K.:   Psychopathic States, New York, 1939, W. W. Norton
      & Co., Inc.
Kahn, Eugen: Psychopathic Personalities, translated by H. Flanders
      Dunbar, New Haven, 1931, Yale University Press.

Questions for Chapter XXIII
Psychopathic Personality

1. What are the characteristics of a person with psychopathic personality?
2. What other terms are sometimes used to designate psychopathic personalities?
3. How is the mental capacity necessarily affected in these patients?
4. What are signs of impending psychopathic personality in adolescents?
5. What are some behavior patterns which psychopathic personalities may
   follow?
6. What are the reasons for antisocial behavior?
7. What is the expectancy for recovery for these patients?
8. Would you expect these persons to learn by experience?
9. Why do these patients usually prove trouble-makers when incarcerated?

Psychopathos

I Emotional Instability.
II Inadequate Personality — Like an overgrown child.
III Paranoid Personality — Persecution
IV Psychopathic Vagabonds —
V Pathological liar - Trait
VI Perverts

CHAPTER XXIV

THE PSYCHONEUROSES

The psychoneuroses are among the most complex, variable and yet most interesting afflictions of mankind. They are responsible for a great deal of human misery but are regarded as being rather benign, for they do not cause a serious disorganization of personality as do the true psychoses. While a psychosis involves the total fabric of personality, according to Meyer, the psychoneurosis is only a part-reaction.

A psychoneurosis is a form of nervousness with various bodily disturbances none of which have an organic basis but which are really outward manifestations of a mental conflict, the exact nature of which the patient is not immediately aware.

The terms neurosis and psychoneurosis practically mean one and the same thing, but some prefer to apply the former to a true physical exhaustion of the nervous system, while the latter is more strictly a form of nervousness based on a psychological disturbance.

In general a psychoneurotic person is excessively aware of his bodily functions and of any sensory experiences which arise therefrom. Moreover, this awareness of self is disagreeable and demands a certain priority in consciousness. There is a strong desire to discuss these physical or bodily tensions, to constantly seek for assurance and for some kind of treatment.

These disturbances are real, not imaginary. The physician and the nurse must continually resist the temptation to look upon psychoneurotic patients as being wilfully sick; their troubles are as strange and undesir-

able a visitation upon them as is a skin rash or an attack
of pneumonia. The psychoneurotic is keenly aware of
his illness as it expresses itself in terms of physical discomfort, but he has little or no knowledge of the true
basis of his symptoms.

Causes of Psychoneurosis.—The source of the trouble
is said to be in the less conscious or in the unconscious
phases of mind in the form of a mental conflict. So far
no other explanation has been as practical or feasible.
This conflict is one between two or more divergent instinctual trends or desires. The symptoms of nervousness arise to consciousness because of an inability to
effect a compromise between these clashing desires. The
nervous state represents a flight from these troublesome
mental tensions into a state of physical illness which is
perforce functional and not organic. Each inner drive
or innate trend is represented usually by a group of
ideas which are held together by a strong emotional
bond or common feeling and is known as a *complex*.
Each complex demands free expression in conscious activity, and in attempting such free expression it may be
working at cross purposes with another complex which
is equally demanding. Thus one often senses in a psychoneurotic patient a struggle between the desire to express sex satisfactions on the one hand and to retain
social and conventional approbation on the other. In
other words, a war exists between the sex urge and the
herd instinct.

The majority of people carry on well enough by various unconscious strategies or compromises. It is here
where many of the mental dynamisms discussed in a
previous chapter come into play. In those cases where
the personality is inherently weak or where the conflict
is one between drives which are more or less evenly

matched, there is the temptation to ease the stress by converting the mental problem unwittingly into physical illness.

Classification of the Psychoneuroses.—There is no universally accepted classification of the psychoneuroses largely because the symptoms of one often overlap the symptoms of another. The simplest clinical grouping which enjoys the greatest popularity is that of Freud.

1. *Neurasthenia,* a simple nervous exhaustion where physical and mental fatigue and general irritability are the outstanding symptoms.

2. *Anxiety state,* a condition where a general fear state is associated with alarming bodily symptoms which produce a sense of impending physical disaster.

3. *Psychasthenia,* a nervous condition marked by an obsessive preoccupation with a single idea or act, usually of a trivial nature and against the patient's better judgment.

4. *Hysteria,* a unique mental state wherein mental tension and anxiety over a personal problem are usually displaced by prominent, disabling physical defects, simulating some true disease and serving a definite purpose, but such purpose is not consciously entertained by the patient.

Neurasthenia

The term neurasthenia, which was introduced by Beard in 1880, is loosely applied to all mild forms of psychoneurosis. Specifically it consists in a great sense of fatigue, associated with marked irritability, an aversion to noise and commotion, insomnia, preoccupation with vague aches and pains and some difficulty in concentration and memory. Marked lassitude particularly during the morning hours is a prominent feature.

Overwork and excessive mental activity are popularly believed to be a prime etiological factor. Freud expressed the opinion that neurasthenic symptoms may be due to excessive masturbation. A careful analysis usually reveals some trying emotional situation which has been repressed and converted into physical debility. Probably behind all these exciting causes one can always detect a fundamental constitution with a strong disposition to easy mental fatigue.

Anxiety State

Anxiety state is probably the most frequent psychoneurosis encountered in private practice. The patient with this form of nervousness consults many physicians and changes from one form of treatment to another at frequent intervals. He is particularly fond of describing his feelings in detail and expresses many apprehensions about the outcome. He is usually of the belief that his ailment is a rare one which the physician cannot understand or cure. This encourages the erroneous impression that he enjoys his illness, but actually the desire for medical attention is simply a part of his illness. The physical symptoms are numerous but generally center about the vital organs of the body. This constant preoccupation with organs which the patient believes are diseased is called *hypochondriasis*. "I feel a tightness in my stomach." "My heart beats fast, and I feel as if it might suddenly stop." "I have no appetite." "My bowels are very loose, and my abdomen feels very heavy." These are frequent complaints offered by the patient. Palpitation, a feeling of suppression of breathing, compression sensations in the head, tight sensations in the throat, numbness in the extremities, as well as a constant feeling of exhaustion are other typical experiences enumerated by the victim of anxiety psychoneurosis. These usually frighten the patient; he cannot concentrate on his work, feels depressed, and harbors fears of sudden death or insanity. Frequently many of these symptoms seize upon the patient at once, throwing him into a panic of acute fear. He dreads being left alone, clings to his family, avoids crowds and public places because he anticipates some dreadful form of collapse.

The fundamental cause of the anxiety state probably lies in the hereditary constitution and in a predisposition to excessive worry over minor physical irregularities. The exciting causes are those based on some threat to self-security, some insult to pride and self-esteem, such as fear of sexual impotence, domestic friction, loss of position, or fear of poverty. Some authorities are particularly prone to emphasize the sexual sources, and Freud expressed the opinion that coitus interruptus was the most common underlying source of the anxiety.

The main features of this psychoneurosis will be found in the following case report.

B. G., a male aged 34 years, was referred to the clinic because he was nervous, could not sleep, and had a peculiar "gone feeling" in his chest. He was a bank teller and had been married three years.

His trouble began some three months before. One morning while working at his window at the bank he suddenly became weak, his heart rate became rapid, his hands began to tremble, and he perspired freely; the thought overwhelmed him that he was about to die. He retired to the employees' rest room and a physician was called. The latter assured him he was not in critical condition, gave him some sedative tablets, and advised him to stay home and rest for two weeks.

After this rest he was no better. He became acutely aware of his heart beat and suffered from pressure sensations in the temples "as if his head were in a vise." He insisted on consulting a heart specialist who found no evidence of organic disease. To his wife he expressed the fear of "something snapping in his head" and causing insanity. He dreaded going out of the house; on finding himself in a crowd his symptoms became worse. His wife, to distract him from his troubles, induced him to go to a movie; in a few minutes he began to perspire, his vision blurred, and in a panic he left the theater.

He returned to work but could scarcely "finish out the day." His head pressure became worse and at the time he was interviewed he cautiously inquired whether he might not have a brain tumor and requested an x-ray examination of the head.

The physical examination was essentially negative. His pupils were dilated. The skin was slightly flushed about the face; there was increased perspiration in the armpits, in the palms, and over the feet. Reflexes were all exaggerated, but no abnormal responses were observed.

In the psychiatric interview the patient admitted that he was a chronic worrier. He was of a German family whose culture and habits were not like those of his associates at the bank. While he was very much attached to his parents, he was rather ashamed of some of their social customs. He married a girl who was of English stock and whose parents did not approve of his background. The latter pointedly refused his frequent invitations to visit his own parents. This worried him greatly, but he rarely discussed the matter openly with his wife. Occasionally he requested her to look up some recipes for some of his favorite German dishes which his mother had been accustomed to prepare. This she evaded doing, and he became very angry because he felt that her mother had influenced her in her bias against German food. Moreover, the patient offered the opinion that his wife was frigid and indifferent. He often found himself entertaining the feeling that he was an "outsider" in his own home.

The nervous condition was undoubtedly the result of his domestic difficulties. His physical symptoms were the result of repressed feelings with a conversion of his tension into fears of heart disease and insanity.

He required frequent assurance and a number of interviews before he was able to discuss his family troubles freely. It was clearly explained to him that he must not rely on medication for relief and that his recovery depended on a rational solution of his family problems. His attacks of anxiety gradually decreased in frequency and severity.

Hysteria

Hysteria as a disturbance in the rational behavior of man was known since the time of the Greek era of medicine. The word is derived from the Greek *hystera,* meaning the womb, for the physicians of ancient times believed the disease was due to the uterus wandering about within the body. In medieval times the person with hysteria was thought to be possessed by demons. The French clinicians of a century ago found that they could induce hysteric symptoms in appropriate subjects at will through suggestion and hypnosis. Attracted by the French clinics and their interest in nervous diseases, Freud went to Paris in 1890 and began his far-reaching investigations into the psychoneuroses. He studied a young girl with hysterical paralysis and concluded that the symptoms could be traced back to some psychic shock of a sexual nature which the patient suffered in early childhood. The memory of this disagreeable event was forgotten or repressed, only to appear later disguised as a physical symptom. Hence the term *conversion hysteria.*

Hysteria is a purposeful, although unconscious psychological mode of reaction by which the patient utilizes a physical symptom as a disguise in order that some acute problem may be solved or some desire fulfilled, the open or conscious gratification of which is shameful to the individual. Hysteria represents a primitive, instinctual mechanism to which a person resorts when he is incapable of adjusting himself through the usual methods of sensible deliberation and rational volitional activity.

We find that hysteria tends to develop in young persons and adults in whom one can sense a childish, naïve, emotionally immature constitutional background. Individuals with hysterical personalities are vain and selfish and like to be the center of attraction. They are apt to be dramatic, abnormally suggestible, even though on the surface they may be intellectually bright and imaginative. This vivid imagination tends to run in the direction of romantic phantasies that possess the immature qualities of those of a boy or girl in the years of

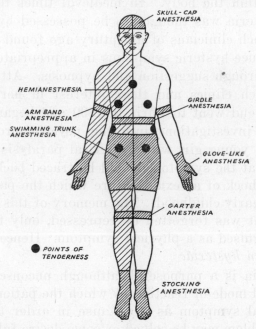

SKULL-CAP
ANESTHESIA

HEMIANESTHESIA

GIRDLE
ANESTHESIA

ARM BAND
ANESTHESIA

SWIMMING TRUNK
ANESTHESIA

GLOVE-LIKE
ANESTHESIA

GARTER
ANESTHESIA

● POINTS OF
TENDERNESS

STOCKING
ANESTHESIA

Fig. 31.—The common forms of sensory disturbance in hysteria. The areas are the result of suggestion and conform to the distribution of wearing material. Painful spots are usually over some vital organ.

puberty. A healthy adult sexuality is lacking in these people. They are said to be arrested at a narcissistic level.

Hysteria can resemble practically every infirmity which is capable of making a strong emotional impression on another individual. The hysterical person unconsciously selects a dramatic set of symptoms which are dictated by suggestion or by having had some previous acquaintance with people who had genuine disease. Hence paralysis, blindness, stupor, epilepsy, and mental blankness are afflictions commonly presented by the victim of hysteria. The symptoms presented in hysteria may therefore be either physical or mental.

Sensory disturbances are unique in that they do not follow the distribution of a nerve but correspond to the patient's own concept of nerve disease, conforming to a functional unit such as the arm, the leg or one-half of the body. Frequently the "numb" areas are suggested by the position of a certain garment on the body as the glove, the stocking, an arm band, etc. In spite of these areas of total numbness to pain or any sensation in the hands, the patient may be able to manipulate a coin in a natural manner. When blindness is claimed, the patient usually avoids obstructions in his path.

Motor disturbances are usually alarming on first appearance. One arm, one side of the body, or both legs may be paralyzed, and this paralysis may be either flaccid or spastic. The legs may be distorted in froglike fashion or may be extremely flexed so that the knees almost touch the chin. Occasionally an hysteric patient develops a loss of vocal cord activity and cannot talk, a condition known as aphonia.

Mental changes characteristic of hysteria are always startling. The patient may go into trancelike states and appear to be utterly oblivious to his surroundings, lying quietly in bed and responding not at all to any painful stimuli. This condition is termed *catalepsy*. Again in some patients there is a predisposition to violent motor reactions simulating an epileptic fit. The patient falls down with a dramatic commotion of writhing and screaming, stiffens the body, holds the breath until the face is blue, and then thrashes the limbs about. Rarely

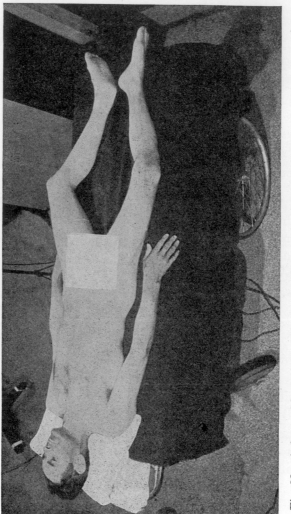

Fig. 32.—A form of hysterical paralysis simulating the position of the posterior limbs of a frog.

does the individual hurt himself in spite of the apparent violence, and the tongue is never bitten as it is in true epilepsy. The hysterical fit almost always occurs in the presence of others and promptly ceases if the patient is left alone. Moreover, there is none of the confusion or stupor which ordinarily follows the genuine epileptic attack.

Another hysterical mental phenomenon is *fugue* or *hysterical amnesia*. The patient obliterates recollection of certain periods of time or certain situations which are associated with great fear or shameful humiliation. Thus the hysteric person conveniently forgets his identity, fails to recognize his relatives and his home environment, or wanders off to a distant city apparently with the selective purpose of "getting away" from his distress and appealing to the sympathy and intriguing the curiosity and aid of strangers.

Whatever the physical disabilities may be in hysteria, a characteristic feature of them all is the attitude of indifference which the patient entertains toward his handicaps. There seems to be a peculiar air of contentment about the patient with hysterical paralysis. He seems to be more relieved than distressed, an attitude which at once suggests that the patient prefers physical defect to mental torment.

Special forms of hysteria can develop and spread as a peculiar form of contagion in large groups of people. Observations have been made of people during an earthquake, in theater fires, and in mob activity. In the panics which ensue from such catastrophes, the behavior of the single individual has the characteristic instinctual and primitive defense reactions which belong to the hysterical phenomenon. Individuals in panic either run about in violent, aimless fashion or fall down in trembling paralysis. In the last world war many soldiers anticipating injury and sudden death became mute and motionless after the explosion of a shell in the immediate vicinity. This severe form of hysteria was called *shell shock* and is now recognized as a more or less unsuccessful attempt to repress the instinct of self-preservation.

The case of a patient with hysteria is presented to illustrate some of the important features of this interesting psychoneurosis:

F. H., a young man 22 years of age, was admitted to the hospital because he had lost his voice. He communicated with the physician and nurses quite willingly by answering all questions with a pencil and pad. He submitted the information that he had not been able to talk for several weeks, that one morning after a sleepless night, he found himself unable to utter a sound. He denied any trouble or emotional tension about home affairs except to state that he was very much concerned about his mother and insisted that she be allowed to visit him every day.

From his mother it was learned that he had always been a lively, imaginative boy who was very sensitive, demanded a great deal of his parents' attention and had frequent temper tantrums if he was crossed in any manner. When the patient was 14 years old, his father was killed in an auto accident. On returning from the funeral, the boy disappeared from home and was found wandering about the streets of a small town forty miles from home. He had taken with him his accordion, which he professed he could not play, nor could he explain to the police who found him just how he came to possess it.

Three years before his admission his mother married a second time. Again he disappeared and was apprehended in a tourist train which was bound for the northwest states.

In recent months he became restless and irritable because he felt that his stepfather was abusing his mother. Three weeks before, he came home one evening to find his parents engaged in a minor argument over household bills. The patient suddenly exploded with a loud denunciation of his stepfather. The latter retaliated by threatening to throw him out of the house and told him he did not want to "hear a sound" from him again. The following morning the patient became mute.

In the hospital he was found to have no physical explanation for his vocal paralysis. His respirations were normal, and he was able to cough without difficulty. One day while in the recreation room with a group of other patients, he overheard an altercation between two of them. Without warning he fell to the floor, seized a rug between his teeth, and with one hand grasped the ankle of a patient and proceeded to jerk his own body about in a thrashing manner. Attempts on the part of attendants to control him only served to increase his strength and violence. It required a general anesthetic to free his hold on the very much frightened fellow patient.

He continued to be mute until one evening he suddenly welcomed the night nurse with a "Hello." This nurse had been unusually interested in his affliction, had granted him some small favors, and had allowed him to assist her in ruling ward charts and keeping temperature records. Thereafter his ability to speak was entirely normal, and a few days later he was discharged.

Psychasthenia

Psychasthenia is a term introduced by the French physician Janet. Literally it means "weakness of the spirit," but actually it is applied to all those nervous reactions characterized by phobias, obsessions, and compulsions. The psychasthenic person is one who is driven to think about or to do something which he recognizes as being senseless or foolish. There is an excessive preoccupation with a single idea or a compulsion to carry out and to repeat over and over again certain acts against his better judgment.

Back of these compulsive or obsessive states is a personality which is by nature conscience-driven, sensitive, shy, strait-laced, fussy, meticulous and precise about bodily functions, dress, religious duty, and daily routine.

Intellectually patients with psychasthenia are generally above average, but their total accomplishment may not be great because of their continual preoccupation with small imperfections. They are tormented by doubts and indecisions over matters which are of little concern to the normal person and cling to others for conviction and reassurance. The prim school girl and the meticulous woman who is passing through the menopause are the most frequent victims of psychasthenia, although it appears in both sexes at any time of life. Usually the psychoneurosis is present in a mild form for many years before it finally becomes a "gnawing, tormenting urgency." A harmless repetition of certain little acts or the persistent recurrence of some senseless thought in consciousness are minor forms of this neurosis. Cracks in the sidewalk are carefully counted, and the individual avoids stepping on them. Doors must be checked two or three times, to make sure that they are locked for the night. Water faucets are reinspected over and over again for leakage before the patient can retire free of tension. Occasionally the individual broods over slight misdemeanors in the remote past or is possessed by ideas which are malicious and vulgar. This induces a great sense of guilt. "Why did I not correct that man when he used obscene language? I now feel that by not doing so I have blasphemed God." "When I told my teacher I had completed my theme, I lied. Why did I do it?" Such retrospections are repeated over and over again, no matter how often friends and relatives reassure the patient that there is no occasion for such abnormal concern.

Psychasthenia is a serious nervous illness because the imperative ideas so control the patient that he becomes a slave to his morbid preoccupation and can scarcely carry on his normal work and social activity. Dominating fears or *phobias* are the most outstanding feature of psychasthenia. The patient fears dirt, bacteria, cancer, and insanity. There may be a senseless fear of open places, of narrow corridors and small rooms, of running water, of staircases, of high places, and of various animals. In fact the phobia may be focused on anything which in some manner suggests death, disease, or disaster.

This senseless fear which is so characteristic of the sensitive, scrupulous-minded individual is probably one which rises out of the unconscious levels because of strong repression of certain disagreeable and shameful feelings. Instead of an open anxiety or frank expression of some instinctual desires, the ideas and intense emotions attached to them are forced out of consciousness. Such pent-up emotional energy attaches itself to an entirely different idea or activity and forces itself into consciousness as a strange tension which has little or no relationship to the original idea. Throughout all these obsessive formations there is sensed a feeling of guilt; the dominating idea seems to become a temptation which the patient must resist by scrupulous conduct. There is a sense of relief after performing the compulsive act, as if a crime had been paid for with an appropriate self-punishment. The neurosis, therefore, is an example of displacement and symbolization; the original conflict with selfish or shameful desires is replaced by a tension over some less disgusting idea or temptation presenting itself as a symbol. Just how this displacement of conflict actually occurs is only theoretically understood. An example of a very pronounced psychasthenic state is demonstrated in the following case report.

H. B., a man 47 years old, presented his problem at the dispensary after he had had a rest cure in a private sanitarium for three months.

During his college days he had had a minor nervous breakdown due to excessive worry about self-abuse. His pastor had been consulted, and after several conferences he was able to resume his school work and graduated at the age of twenty-one years as an accountant. He admitted that he was always very conscientious, worried a great deal about body cleanliness, and was known for his finicky desire to keep his room and clothing in perfect order. He was always prompt in appearing at his office and never left his desk before five o'clock. His fellow workers regarded him as very fussy and his employer always remarked about the neatness of his desk and files—a comment which greatly pleased him. At home any irregularity in household routine upset him very badly. His wife was fully aware of his rigid regard for rules and of his scrupulousness.

Four months before the present interview he was assigned the rather formidable task of making out the income tax report for his firm, which dealt in stocks and bonds. This assignment was made on March 1, and he realized that he had but two weeks before the returns were to be filed. He worked under great pressure and almost every day he remained in the office until late at night. With a day to spare, he entered the final figures on a roll from an adding machine. Badly lacking sleep and rest, he seized this roll, thrust it into his overcoat pocket, and dashed for the midnight street car to his home. He had intended to show the slip of paper to his wife as evidence that his job was completed. On his arrival at his home he could not find the roll. In a frenzy he searched his clothing, ran out on the street searching the sidewalk, but failed to find it. He was put to bed in a badly agitated condition and remained under a physician's care for several weeks.

On returning to work, he found himself a prey to a peculiar compulsion. He could no longer pass a piece of crumpled paper on the floor or sidewalk without picking it up and inspecting it. During rush hour he was greatly humiliated and embarrassed by the necessity of bending over and picking up odd bits of paper. On several occasions during this performance he was knocked down by hurrying passersby. A wastebasket full of discarded paper literally threw him into a panic. His only relief was obtained by waiting after office hours and going over each item piece by piece. A visit to a sanitarium was recommended. There he became considerably better, but the obsessive idea remained, and for this reason he came to the dispensary. He was well oriented, intelligent, had good insight, and otherwise was mentally normal.

Behind this obsessive tension state was obviously a sensitive, overconscientious personality. Possibly the basic trouble was a sexual difficulty. His wife furnished the information that he never was very virile in his sex life and seemed to be indirectly aware of this failing. However, because of his fastidious nature, she rarely mentioned the matter, and he avoided any discussion of it.

Compulsive behavior and obsessive fears are substitution devices which relieve tension arising out of a sense of guilt or a feeling of personal insecurity. Unfortunately the relief offered by the act is only temporary and the ritual must be repeated at frequent intervals. Relatives lose patience and attempt to "break the patient of his habit." This only causes the victim to become restless, uncomfortable and agitated, for the act has become a fixed channel for the discharge of all tension due to innate instinctual conflict. Psychasthenia is one of the most stubborn of all the psychoneuroses; it may improve for a period of time, but in many patients it remains a constant feature of the personality. In those most unfortunate persons in whom the obsessive tension is such that total incapacity exists for years, the operation called prefrontal lobotomy may offer considerable relief if not actual recovery.

War Neuroses. There is no great difference between peace and war neuroses, but individual patterns of neurotic behavior give way to mass reactions which are of an hysterical nature. In the civilian population, war arouses fear regarding the safety of the community because of risk of attack, because of economic changes, threat of family separation and threat of food shortage. When such tensions in the general population occur, there is a tendency to false rumor, to great suggestibility and to relief of nervousness through lowered moral behavior and, in certain unstable persons, to delinquency, petty crime, and other abnormal aggressive behavior.

Observation on soldiers in active duty reveals every type of neurotic disturbance. Men with previous anxiety symptoms, depressed, sensitive, timorous and phobic individuals are usually unable to stand the strain of war, and the condition is usually rapidly aggravated within a few weeks after entering military service. In the more stable soldier, the terrifying experiences of actual combat, physical and mental fatigue, exposure to weather, loss of sleep, lack of food or water, may lead to severe neurotic symptoms, many of which, however, may disappear after an appropriate period of complete rest. The chronic and permanent neuroses are found usually in the soldier whose pre-existing personality was poorly balanced and adjusted. Shell shock is no longer regarded as an adequate term for these acute mental and nervous reactions to military experience: "combat fatigue" is found to be more inclusive and descriptive.

Treatment of the Psychoneuroses.—The multitude of theories and methods of handling psychoneurotic patients is bewildering. Only a few of the more common principles can be discussed here. It can be said that back of all psychoneuroses is a feeling of inferiority, an excess of ambition, or an inability to endure failures. Hence the physician and the nurse should "see around" the immediate physical symptoms which are thrust at one and sense the real trouble behind them. To treat the physical complaints with medication is only leading the patient deeper into his neurosis. Unfortunately, this is the very course which many unwary physicians pursue. It serves only to make the nervous disorder a chronic one, for the physician soon learns that the more medicine administered the more chronic and stubborn the symptoms become.

Psychotherapy is a more rational form of treatment because it seeks the very source of the disorder. *Psychotherapy* is any procedure which promotes the development of courage, inner security, and self-confidence.

It may be anything from a pat on the back to an elaborate mental analysis requiring several years. The most effective methods in psychotherapy are suggestion, analysis, and re-education. It consists of an effort to teach the patient to understand himself, the particular nature of his illness, and how his physical troubles are caused by the deeper problems of his mental life. Psychotherapy is not a fixed technique; it is more an art than a science, and its methods must be adapted and modified to fit the individual situation. In plain language it is a form of mental exploration. The important steps may be presented as follows:

1. The patient must have confidence in the physician and some respect for his knowledge and experience. A word of assurance alone may be the deciding factor in relieving many psychoneurotics of their forebodings and anxieties. Such a relationship is regarded as a satisfactory *rapport*.

2. The patient is simply encouraged to talk about his life experiences. His tongue is allowed to run on, wherever it will, as long as he relates his own memories. This random talk will allow the patient freely to follow the associations in his mind and is in substance a kind of *mental ventilation*. The trained physician will note that there are certain occasions and events which the patient dismisses quickly or avoids mentioning except in a slurring way.

3. These "sore points" are then discussed with greater frankness. The patient is encouraged to talk about them more freely until they no longer cause excess emotion, a process known as *desensitization*.

4. The patient is then acquainted with the manner in which his repressed feelings produced his condition. This should be done in a simple, clear style, thereby

teaching the patient to gain insight into the exact nature of his illness. Thus begins the process of *re-education*.

5. The subject is then encouraged to face his distressing troubles, and, instead of running away from them, he is urged to think of them, not to "forget" them, to become familiar with them, and to approach their solution in a candid, open manner.

During and after such a psychotherapeutic program, the patient should be given every opportunity to rest, to correct bad habits of working, eating, and exercising. The rest cure in a sanatorium is an excellent opportunity for correcting these faulty habits, but it must be emphasized that such a treatment does not in itself offer a cure but is merely an aid in restoring normal physical vitality. If this explanation is not made, the psychoneurotic person frequently uses the hospital as another refuge from his mental conflicts and may become an "addict" to institutional life.

Psychoanalysis.—Psychoanalysis is a formidable discipline or technique introduced by Sigmund Freud, which allows a very exhaustive mental exploration in those situations where the simpler and less formal methods do not seem to uncover the cause. It is fundamentally a method of exploring the unconscious mind where are imbedded the sources of mental illness. The main features of this impressive method of mental treatment are the interesting devices by which mental conflicts are probed for in the unconscious layers of the mind and are brought to conscious levels. The analyst at first strives for this objective by means of *free association*. This consists mainly of noting the spoken thoughts of patients when they are off guard or when they make random remarks during periods of absent-mindedness. Another device is one in which the patient is given a list of words and is asked to respond with any idea which the particular word provokes. Words which bring forth painful associations are followed by a delay in response, that is, the association time is prolonged. From a systematic perusal of words which apparently induced disturbing and hesitant responses, the analyst can often obtain a lead as to the basic problem.

In some psychoneuroses, particularly hysteria, the repressed material can be made accessible by *hypnosis*. This consists of inducing by suggestion a state of unconsciousness or sleep, during which the patient will unknowingly disclose forgotten memories and freely answer questions relating to his true wishes or desires. Hypnosis is not, however, regarded as a technique in psychoanalysis.

Another technique which the analyst utilizes is to look into the substance of dreams, for dreams are considered wish-fulfilling realizations of unconscious cravings. But these desires present themselves in the dream disguised as symbols or condensations, for they are not permitted to appear in their true form. It is the function of the analyst to re-interpret these in their true light.

As this ventilation proceeds and the patient becomes aware of the true nature of his strivings and conflicts, he unconsciously focuses his liberated libido forces upon the physician. The critical point is the physician's ability to disperse this psychic energy into useful and more natural social channels. This brings into play the process of *sublimation*.

Psychoanalysis is a venture with unpredictable results. In some neuroses it appears to do more harm than good. Some authorities wholeheartedly denounce psychoanalysis. Its full application should be left to those who have had special experience with its correct management.

The Nursing Care of Psychoneurotic Patients.—In no other disorder is it so important for the nurse to maintain a strictly objective attitude toward the patient and his symptoms. The psychoneurotic individual is unconsciously driven by his physical troubles to complain, to get attention, and to demand treatment. The line of least resistance is to sympathize openly and to give in to little demands. This is obviously wrong. The correct attitude is to keep in mind the true factor behind the symptoms, to avoid discussing them, and to lead the patient's interest away from his introspections into healthy, constructive activities, both mental and physical. Even such supporting treatment as hydrotherapy, massage, and heat may be accepted by the neurotic patient as confirming evidence that he is physically sick, and they should be applied with great discretion. Occupational therapy, on the other hand, is of prime importance for it enhances self-respect, stimulates creative ability, and promotes self-reliance. Naturally, a psychoneurotic patient may develop true physical illness as any other human being may do. Hence it is necessary for the nurse to be acquainted with the common complaints of the psychoneurotic patient so that they can be readily separated from symptoms which indicate serious organic trouble.

The nurse should resist the temptation to scorn the psychoneurotic as being a weakling or an impostor. He is always to be given consideration which is neither too cool or too patronizing, on the one hand, nor too sentimental and indulgent, on the other.

References

Culpin, Millais: Recent Advances in the Study of the Psychoneuroses, Philadelphia, 1931, P. Blakiston's Son & Co.
Emerson, Charles P.: The Nervous Patient, Philadelphia, 1935, J. B. Lippincott Company.

Freud, Sigmund: Studies in Hysteria, translated by A. A. Brill, New
    York, Nervous and Mental Disease Monographs.
Glover, Edward: An Investigation of the Technique of Psychoanalysis,
    Baltimore, 1940, Williams & Wilkins Co.
Kardiner, Abram: The Traumatic Neuroses of War, New York, 1941,
    Paul B. Hoeber, Inc.
Kretschmer, Ernst: Hysteria, translated by Oswald H. Boltz, New York,
    1926, Nervous and Mental Disease Publishing Co.
Miller, Emanuel: The Neuroses in War, New York, 1940, The Macmillan
    Co.
Rixon and Matthew: Anxiety Hysteria, New York, 1921, Paul B.
    Hoeber.
Wechsler, I. S.: The Neuroses, Philadelphia, 1939, W. B. Saunders
    Company.

Questions for Chapter XXIV

The Psychoneuroses

1. Explain the definition of psychoneurosis.
2. How do some people distinguish between neurosis and psychoneurosis?
3. Are psychoneurotic symptoms real or imaginary? Is the patient a malingerer?
4. Define "complex." What do you understand by "mental conflict"?
5. What are the outstanding symptoms of neurasthenia?
6. Describe a typical patient with an anxiety state.
7. What is hypochondriasis? Give examples.
8. Explain psychasthenia.
9. Describe the hysterical personality.
10. Do hysterical patients show only physical symptoms?
11. List some of the symptoms which patients with hysteria may show.
12. What are the determinative symptoms?

CHAPTER XXV

PHYSICAL THERAPY

Therapy by the application of various physical agents such as manual massage, electricity, light, heat, and water has been developed in recent years as a systematized specialty. When these methods of treatment were first introduced, many sweeping and unwarranted claims were made as to their value. They were used indiscriminately in a wide range of physical ailments. As experience accumulated and expert training in physical therapy became available, a more rational and restricted application was made of these procedures, and at the present time physical therapy rests on a sound and scientific basis.

Only those techniques which find an immediate and positive value in the treatment of mental and nervous disorders can be presented in this discussion.

Hydrotherapy—Water is essentially a useful physical agent in treatment because of its capacity to convey heat into or out of the body of the patient. In psychiatry, baths of different types affect the nervous system indirectly by producing changes in the pulse, blood pressure, respiration and in the body temperature. It is possible that water also has a direct psychological effect on the patient, but just how this occurs cannot be clearly demonstrated.

The Continuous Tub Bath

This treatment has a sedative effect upon a large percentage of noisy, restless patients. It also serves to keep the destructive and untidy patient under very close supervision and away from others who are not so disturbed.

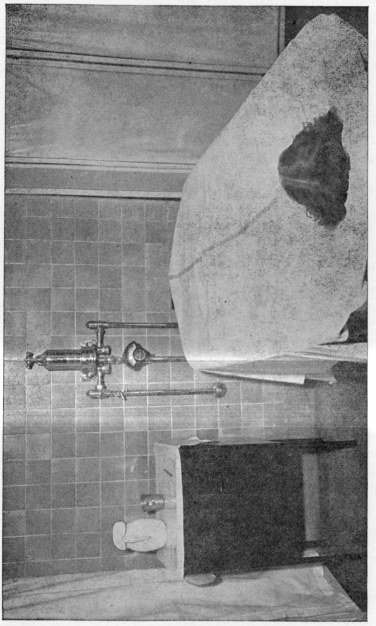

Fig. 33.—The continuous tub bath. Only the head of the patient is exposed above the canvas cover. The mixing chamber for regulating the water temperature is shown attached to the wall.

The tubs are specially constructed so that a continuous inflow and outflow of water take place. The patient rests on a canvas hammock which is suspended in the water. Over the patient is placed a canvas cover which is fastened to the side bars of the tub.

The tub should be in readiness to receive the patient, with the hammock and cover in place and the water circulating at a level sufficient to keep the body completely immersed. The temperature of the water should be about 94° or 95° F. The patient's body is covered with a thin film of olive or mineral oil, or petrolatum, and the patient is then quickly placed in the tub with as little confusion as possible. Ample help should be at hand, and the tub cover is placed over the patient immediately and fastened securely to the tub. Knots should not be tied in the fastenings as it may be necessary to remove the cover quickly in an emergency. The fastenings are to be wound around the bars provided for this purpose. A rubber pillow provides a rest for the patient's head.

The tub room is kept as quiet as possible with no more lights, noise, or conversation than necessary. The patient's pulse is taken and charted every fifteen minutes. The temperature of the water is tested both by the immersed hand and a reliable thermometer set in a wooden case. The pulse and the water temperature should be checked more frequently if the patient shows any signs of discomfort. The tub room should never be left unattended, and the nurse's attention is to be devoted exclusively to her patients. Drinking water should be offered the patient at frequent intervals, and cold compresses should be applied to the forehead of the excessively restless patients. At intervals of three or four hours it may be necessary to apply another coating of oil to the patient's skin. Patients can be spoon fed from trays placed on the canvas covers. Continuous tub therapy can be prolonged to as much as eight or ten hours.

The floors of the tub room should be kept dry and clean of debris. The nurse in charge must be ready at an instant's notice to shut off the water and to remove the . patient from the tub. This action is necessary if the patient's color becomes pale, if there is marked irregularity in the pulse rate, if there is an accident to the plumbing, or if the mixing chambers do not function properly. Finally, one must not overlook the possibility of accidental or intentional drowning.

After the continuous bath, the tub is drained; the patient is removed, dried thoroughly, wrapped in warm covers, and placed in a warmed bed.

The Sitz Bath

This treatment, very efficacious in applying external heat to the pelvic region, is administered by requiring the patient to immerse the buttocks and thighs in a specially constructed tub while the feet are immersed in a foot pan.

Articles required are a T binder, sheets, blanket, material for cold compresses, drinking water, foot pan, and thermometer.

Procedure.—The nurse undresses the patient and adjusts the T binder. The sitz tub should be ready, with the water at the prescribed temperature, a folded sheet covering the tub from front to back, and the foot pan filled with water of from 104° to 110° F. The patient is assisted to sit down in the tub, and he is made comfortable, with the sheet covering the back of the tub and arranged so that the legs are not pressed in contact with the front rim of the tub. A sheet plus a blanket, if necessary, is draped completely around the patient and tub, and these coverings are secured with a safety pin.

The sitz bath usually is started at a fairly low temperature which is raised daily until a high degree of heat can be tolerated. The physician will prescribe the duration of the treatment and the degree of heat necessary. The routine sitz bath may be started at 94° F. and raised 2 or 3 degrees every day until a temperature of 106° F. or higher is reached. The average single treatment lasts from three to ten minutes.

The patient should have cold compresses applied to the head during the treatment, and fluids by mouth are given frequently. The nurse should watch for pulse irregularity, headache, or signs of fainting or dizziness and must discontinue the treatment if these occur.

When the treatment is finished, the patient is dried thoroughly, dressed in warm clothing, and allowed to rest before being returned to the ward.

The Cold Wet Sheet Pack

The cold wet sheet pack is one of the most successful methods of controlling the mentally excited patient. At the same time the circulation of the blood and the lymph is improved, elimination is promoted, metabolism is stimulated, and nutrition is heightened. The ultimate results depend upon the extent and character of the patient's reaction to the cold of the moist sheets and the effects obtained from the cold applications to the head.

There are four stages to the cold wet sheet pack, and these must be thoroughly understood by the nurse who has the care of the patient during the treatment, for careful nursing care is of the utmost importance. The patient must understand the nature and purpose of the treatment. It is the nurse's duty to explain this carefully to the patient before the treatment is given.

The first stage is called the cooling or evaporating stage. It lasts from five to twenty minutes, during which time the whole body rallies to resist the cold. The skin becomes pale because the blood vessels of the skin contract and the blood is driven to the internal organs. The patient shivers and gasps with the first contact with the cold sheets. The pulse rate is increased and then becomes full and slower. This stage ends when the temperature of the sheets is raised to normal skin temperature, 92° F. to 94° F. If the patient does not react properly, that is, if he does not produce enough body heat to warm the pack to normal skin temperature, he must be removed, for there is danger of shock. A warm bath and a warm drink should be given. Bed rest with warm blankets and hot water bottles is indicated if the patient fails to warm up. If he fails to become normally warm, friction is applied to the body. Physically healthy persons will react promptly to cold applications.

The second stage is known as the neutral or sedative stage. It begins when the sheets have become as warm as the normal skin temperature. The skin of the body takes on a pinkish hue because the blood vessels of the skin dilate. The color of the face remains normal. A degree of anemia in the brain results. There is a quieting of the general nervous system and a condition conducive to sleep results. To maintain the sedative period, cold compresses may be applied to the head and face, and an ice cap may be put under the neck and head. These are not necessary if the patient is quiet. With proper management this stage may last from three to four hours.

The third stage or heating stage of the cold wet sheet pack begins when the warming of the pack raises the skin temperature above normal. It ends when perspiration begins and the face becomes flushed. The pulse rate increases and becomes less strong. At this time the patient must be removed from the pack.

The fourth stage or sweating stage is not usually used for mental patients. It is used as an eliminative and spoliative measure for certain physical ailments such as nephritis. During this stage perspiration grows profuse, and elevation of temperature occurs. It has a very weakening effect, and care must be used in observation of the pulse and the color and expression of the patient's face. Fluids are given frequently, and cold compresses are applied continuously to the head.

Definition and Purpose.—The sedative cold wet sheet pack is a hydriatic procedure in which the whole body is enveloped, except the head and the soles of the feet, in cold wet sheets and dry blanket covering, so applied as to regulate the evaporation and to produce a sedative effect. It is so applied that no two skin surfaces come in contact.

Articles Required.—(a) Large woolen blanket; (b) two or three moist pack sheets of required temperature, usually about 60° F.; (c) two protecting sheets; (d) sheet for under the head; (e) cover sheet; (f) hot water bottle, 118° F.; (g) basin of iced water; (h) two compress towels; (i) feeding cups; (j) pitcher of water; (k) ice cap; (l) rubber-covered pillow.

Procedure.—All required articles are brought to the bedside.

The blanket is put on the bed with the top edge about ten inches from and parallel with the head rail.

The first sheet is spread over the blanket so that it is just long enough to encapsulate the feet. At the head of the bed the sheet is folded down so that the fold extends 6 inches beyond the upper edge of the blanket.

The arm or cross sheet is folded like a draw sheet and laid across the bed with its fold 6 inches from, and parallel with, the upper edge of the blanket. This sheet must reach from the axillae to below the finger tips.

The nude patient sits and then lies down on the sheets. The fold of the arm sheet must be even with the axillae.

The ends of the arm sheet are brought up between the arm and the body on each side. The patient is turned to the right and the arm sheet smoothed around the left arm and across the back. The arm is extended along the side of the body, care being taken that it is not under the body.

The patient is turned to the left and the sheet smoothed around the right arm and down across the back.

The first sheet is then applied by first pulling the upper right side of the sheet across the patient's chest and abdomen, the upper edge to fit up under the chin. Turn the patient slightly to the right so that the sheet may be smoothed toward the back of the body. The portion of the right side of the sheet which extends below the trunk is brought over the right leg and thigh, and smooth folds are allowed to fall between the legs and thighs.

The left side of the sheet is then brought across the body. A pleat is formed at the right hip. The patient is turned to the right, and the sheet wrapped smoothly and snugly across the patient's back. The lower extremities are enveloped, the soles of the feet being left uncovered.

A hot water bottle at 118° F. is placed at the feet if they are cold.

Now the upper edges of the sheet are smoothed over the shoulders from the back forward and then from the front toward the back. The sheet should fit up under the chin and around the neck to protect the skin from the blanket.

A third sheet, folded to proper size, may be placed over the anterior portion of the trunk. This will help to prolong the sedative stage.

The blanket is applied over the wet sheets in much the same manner as the first sheet. The pleat is omitted as the blanket can be easily made to fit snugly. Envelope folds are made at the shoulders. The blanket extends beyond the feet. It should be folded neatly under the feet.

Protecting sheets, which have been folded diagonally into bands about fifteen inches wide, are applied, one across the chest and one across the knees. These sheets must not be too tight but tight enough to prevent the patient from rolling. They are fastened securely through the side rails.

The head of the mattress is covered with a sheet, and the pack may be covered with a sheet.

If the patient is restless, an ice cap may be placed under the neck and head. The ice cap must not be so full as to cause discomfort.

Cold compresses may be applied to the forehead and face if restlessness occurs during the treatment.

A rubber-covered pillow may be given if the patient is more comfortable with one.

Special care must be taken throughout the application of the pack. There must be no wrinkles. It must fit smoothly and snugly. There is danger of impairing the blood circulation if the sheets are too tight or binding. The pack should be applied quickly.

The nurse should (1) observe the patient closely, take, and record the pulse and respirations every half hour;

(2) Give water when requested;

(3) Keep the room quiet, avoid glaring lights, have the room temperature near 70° F., and keep the air fresh by proper ventilation.

Management of the Patient in the Cold Wet Sheet Pack.—Close observation is imperative. The nurse in charge should be notified if the patient seems not to be reacting properly. Removal of the pack is indicated if the patient shows any of the following signs: (a) Failure to become normally warm within twenty minutes; (b) cyanosis; (c) continued paleness; (d) pulse or respirations above normal; (c) weak pulse; (f) flushed face; (g) perspiration.

The duration of the pack will vary in accordance with the patient's reaction. If each stage of the cold wet pack is properly understood, the nurse will have no difficulty in determining the proper time for discontinuance of the pack.

Charting.—The pulse and respiration are taken and recorded every half hour. The duration and effects of the treatment are charted. The patient's intake is recorded. Bowel movement and frequency of urination should be charted.

Frequency of the Pack.—The doctor specifies the number of treatments. Sometimes several packs are given in a day.

Contraindications.—This treatment is not used unless the patient is in good physical condition. Some of the contraindications are (a) respiratory infection; (b) heart condition; (c) hypertension; (d) senility; (e) inability to react to cold. A cold wet sheet pack is never given without the doctor's written order.

Aftercare.—When removed from the pack, it is well for the patient to go to bed. If the patient is to remain up, he must be dressed warmly and kept in a warm room.

A cleansing tub bath or shower must be given each day. It is important to dry the skin carefully after the bath. Powder or oil may be rubbed gently into the irritated skin areas.

Nourishment.—Liquid nourishment is given while the patient is in the pack. The doctor may order a soft diet when the patient is in the pack at meal time.

Cold Applications to the Head.—When the ice cap or cold compresses are applied to the head, face, or neck, these skin areas must be continuously cold if the proper effect is to be obtained. Therefore, the compresses must be changed frequently. Usually fifteen or twenty minutes of continuous cold application to the head will quiet the patient. These cold applications tend to prevent cerebral congestion, and vital activity is lessened.

The Stimulating Spray

The stimulating spray is an application of many jets of water against the surface of the body from all sides. The initial temperature of the water is 95°-100° F. and should not go below 70° F.

The friction of the water upon the skin stimulates the circulation of the blood. It improves the lymph circulation. Digestion is improved. It restores the tone of the body muscles and other tissues and is conducive to a feeling of well-being.

This treatment is given to those who need improved nutrition and careful stimulation.

Articles Required.—(1) T binder, (2) bathing cap, (3) foot basin of antiseptic solution, (4) towel, (5) talcum powder and cocoa butter.

The temperature of the room should be between 75° F. and 85° F., and the patient should be protected from drafts.

Procedure.—The nurse explains the nature and the purpose of the treatment to the patient. The patient undresses and puts on the T binder and a bathing cap. If the patient is not able to do this, the nurse will do it for her.

The feet are dipped into an antiseptic solution to prevent the spread of foot infection which is common in showers used by more than a few persons.

Then the patient steps into the spray and turns slowly about during the treatment.

When the patient is negativistic, the nurse shall dress in a bathing suit and go into the shower with the patient.

Duration.—The patient remains under the spray for five minutes.

Aftercare.—The body is dried carefully and talcum powder or cocoa butter applied to skin areas which show any irritation.

The Scotch Douche

The Scotch douche may follow the stimulating spray for the purpose of further stimulation.

Procedure.—Hot water at 110° F. and cold water at 80° F. are applied alternately up and down the spine several times.

The water, as it leaves the hose, should be fanned with the finger to prevent striking the patient with too much force.

Duration.—This treatment should not last longer than two minutes.

Aftercare.—Aftercare is the same as that given after the stimulating spray.

Contraindications.—Contraindications to these stimulating treatments are hypertension, respiratory infections, menstruation, and any advanced systemic disease. These treatments are never given without the doctor's written order.

The equipment and floors must be kept very clean. The bathing caps are washed well in soapy water and dried after each patient.

Colonic Irrigation

Definition.—By colonic irrigation the colon is filled and flushed with a large amount of fluid.

Purpose.—It is used to (1) cleanse the colon, (2) relieve irritation, (3) relieve the suppression of urine, (4) induce peristalsis and relieve flatus, (5) relieve toxic conditions, and (6) provide heat.

Requisites.—(1) Tray as for a soapsuds enema, (2) connecting tube, (3) one foot of extra tubing with a clasp, (4) rubber sheet bed protector and cover, (5) two large pitchers of the desired solution at the proper temperature, (6) blanket, (7) standard.

The temperature of the solution should be 100° to 104° F. for cleansing the colon and increasing renal secretion; 104° to 110° F. for disinfection and to relieve visceral pain; or 110° to 116° F. to supply heat in case of shock or collapse. A small soapsuds enema to remove any fecal mass should precede the irrigation.

Position.—The patient may be in the Sims position or in the dorsal position with the hips elevated.

Procedure.—Six inches from the tip the colon tube is marked for insertion into the rectum for inflow. For outflow a colon tube is used one size smaller than the inflow tube. Three inches from the tip the outflow tube is marked for insertion into the rectum; thus the inflow tube is inserted three inches farther than the outflow tube. For convenience the tubes may be held together at the points of marking with a rubber band. One foot of rubber tubing is connected with the outflow tube.

The tubes are lubricated; the air and cold fluid are allowed to escape; the inflow tube is clamped and both tubes are inserted together, allowing the solution to run slowly.

To avoid distressful distention of the colon, the inflow is shut off for a few moments at intervals.

To complete the treatment, the nurse checks the inflow and allows a few minutes for draining the remaining fluid. She then removes the colon tubes, bathes the parts and makes the patient comfortable.

References

Bailey, Harriet: Nursing Mental Diseases, New York, 1934, The Macmillan Company.
Stewart, H. E.: Physiotherapy, Theory and Clinical Application, 2nd edition, New York, 1929, Paul B. Hoeber.
Wright, Rebekah: Hydrotherapy in Hospitals for Mental Diseases, Boston, 1932, The Tudor Press, Inc.

Questions for Chapter XXV
Physical Therapy

1. What is the outstanding property of water that makes it a valuable physical agent?
2. What is the purpose of the continuous tub treatment?
3. In a logical fashion discuss the steps taken in preparation for the treatment.
4. Give the procedure for placing the patient in the tub.
5. Outline the nursing care of the patient during the continuous tub treatment; after the treatment.
6. Enumerate the dangers of the continuous tub treatment.
7. Outline the procedure for the Sitz bath.
8. Describe carefully each of the four stages of the cold wet sheet pack as to physiological action and reaction, duration, and dangers.
9. Give the definition and the purpose of the cold wet sheet pack. What are some other beneficial effects of the cold wet sheet pack?

10. Discuss the management of the wet sheet pack as to the frequency of the treatment, contraindications, charting, nourishment and the signs which indicate removal of the pack.

11. What care must the patient receive after the treatment?

12. What is the purpose of the cold applications to the head? For the proper effect why must they be applied continuously for a given period?

13. Define and give the purpose of the stimulating spray.

14. What beneficial results are derived from the stimulating spray?

15. Discuss the care of the patient before, during, and after the treatment.

16. What is the purpose of the Scotch douche? Discuss the treatment as to method of application, temperatures of water, and duration of treatment. What are the contraindications?

17. What is the purpose of the colonic irrigation? Outline the procedure.

CHAPTER XXVI

OCCUPATIONAL AND RECREATIONAL THERAPY

Nothing has been so effective in relieving the dull tedium of the institution for mental disease as the introduction of occupational and recreational therapy. Young men and women are now being trained in ever increasing numbers to direct their talents and energies in the guiding of the sick and the injured back into creative, health-giving occupation and physical activity.

In occupational therapy, system and precision are as important as in other forms of treatment. It should be prescribed and correlated with other forms of treatment. Less formally it can be applied by the nurse in charge of the ward. The assignment of any of the little manifold tasks in the kitchen, the linen closet, and the utility room of the ward is essentially a form of occupational therapy. The daily performance of some duty in housekeeping, the decoration of the ward for the holidays, assisting the nurse in the chart room—all these are stimulating activities which bring self-security and a sense of usefulness.

In the regularly established department of occupational therapy, the prescribed work is selected with special consideration of the patient's mental condition and native capacity. The work is carried on chiefly in classes or groups so that at the same time social adaptation is encouraged and the patient is stimulated by the example of others. "The goals are to arouse interest, courage, and confidence; to exercise mind and body in healthy activity; to overcome disability and reestablish capacity for industrial and social usefulness.''* Occupational therapy can only be prescribed by order of the physician. The treatment is contraindicated for patients who are suicidal, very untidy, or handicapped by acute physical illness.

The immediate therapeutic value of occupational therapy is diversion of the mental processes from morbid and destructive trends to a wholesome and natural direction. As soon as a patient is able to cooperate, he should be assigned an appropriate activity compatible with his strength and initiative. The nurse can frequently sense from her own observations just what leanings a patient may have and what faculties can be stimulated. The professional occupational therapist is usually adept at observing the spontaneous interests of the new patient and can be guided thereby in outlining a program of work.

The patient may be attracted to work which is new or may prefer to enter into activities with which he is familiar; there is no fixed rule in this respect. Most patients respond to a program which contains some novelty. It is advisable to assign the work in short periods, avoiding long sustained efforts, and, at least in the early phases, to outline a task which can be completed in good time so as to stimulate confidence and a sense of successful accomplishment.

For depressed patients the assignment should be one which does not require prolonged mental effort and which carries with it some simple repetitive maneuver. The hyperactive individual does well in some gross activity such as tearing cloth into strips, where excessive energy can be well dissipated. The brooding and introspective individual should be tested by giving him an assignment which requires a high degree of concentra-

*Rules and Principles of the American Occupational Therapy Association.

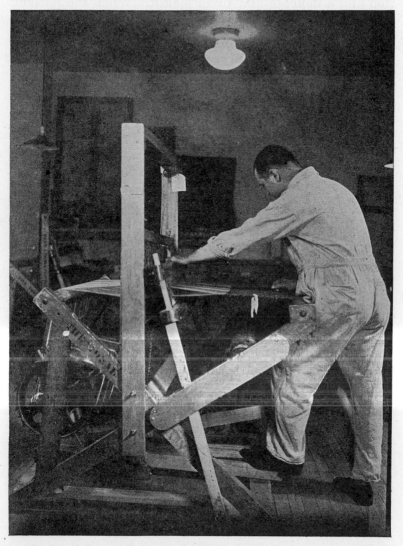

Fig. 34.—In the loom room of occupational therapy. "The therapeutic objective should be to substitute the strongest normal interests available to overcome phantasy preoccupation." (J. B. Davis: Principles and Practice of Occupational Therapy for the Mentally ill.)

O.T. must have Precision + System

O.T. Has to be ⊙ in pt. ability & interest

tion and a delicate and precise skill. When the patient makes a real effort, but the results are poor, he should nevertheless be praised and encouraged. The program must be progressive and a graduated series of problems should be applied, parallel with the progress and improvement in the patient's mental condition.

The special activities and crafts which have been developed in occupational therapy are endless in number and cannot be fully outlined here. The following are examples of those occupations which have been advantageously applied.

For men: Carpentry, furniture construction and repair, wood carving, jigsaw problems, broom and brush making, carpet weaving, leather work, mechanical drawing, bookbinding, printing, brass and copper metal craft.

For women: Sewing, quilting, bead work, knitting, crocheting, loom work of all types, painting, linoleum-block cutting, hooked rugs, dress design.

Recreational Activity.—Outdoor recreation, group activities, games, contests, music, shows, reading, and cultivation of special talents—all have their place in developing physical and mental security in the mental patient. Physical exercise which is so essential in the patient who is confined in a closed institution can be provided through organized classes in calisthenics. Probably more valuable are physical activities which stimulate interest and attract the patient to spontaneously participate. This can be done through the medium of games such as baseball, tennis, croquet, golf, etc. These more vigorous activities should not be prescribed for the older patients whose endurance may be limited because of chronic cardiovascular disease. Walking and working in the garden are recreations preferred and enjoyed by the sedentary or elderly person. Special gymnastic exercises are indicated for those who have some particular infirmity of body or limb.

Informal recreation on the ward is generally organized by the ward nurse and the degree of good it may do depends directly upon her enthusiasm and ingenuity. In the day room of the ward there should be tables for checkers, cards, dominoes, and other board games.

Reading should be encouraged if the patient cannot indulge in the more active pastimes and particularly if bedridden. Light fiction and biography are preferable. Discourses on religion, psychology, philosophy, and medical matters should be avoided.

Every recreational and occupational activity has a positive value in psychiatry because it serves to relax tension, stimulates self-respect, and above all turns the patient's psychic life into the more healthful interests of the outside world and away from inner, morbid, and disintegrating trends. Even the deteriorated patient shows surprising capacities when participating in simple games or contests, where otherwise the mental faculties become dormant and blunted. Occupational therapy is regarded by some psychiatrists as "the most powerful single means at our command in curative treatment."

References

Davis, John E., in collaboration with Dr. William R. Dunton, Jr.: Principles and Practice of Recreational Therapy for the Mentally Ill, New York, 1936, A. S. Barnes & Co.

Slagle, Eleanor C. (editor): Games and Field Day Programs, Utica, New York, 1933, State Hospitals Press.

Slagle and Robeson: Syllabus for Training of Nurses in Occupational Therapy, Utica, New York, 1933, State Hospitals Press.

Questions for Chapter XXVI

Occupational and Recreational Therapy

1. Distinguish between occupational and recreational therapy.
2. What are some ward activities which can be assigned to patients and which will have a therapeutic value?

3. What is the immediate value of occupational therapy?
4. What points should the nurse observe with patients who are attending occupational therapy classes?
5. What type of therapy usually is prescribed for depressed patients? For manic patients? For schizophrenic patients?
6. What factors should the nurse assisting with recreational therapy for mentally ill patients consider?
7. What are some games which the nurse might organize on the ward?
8. Name some books which could be recommended to mental patients for reading.
9. Plan a holiday party for the patients on your ward, considering decorations, games, and refreshments. Assign patients to certain duties according to their ability and psychological need.

CHAPTER XXVII

SHOCK THERAPY IN MENTAL DISEASE

Because the treatment of certain mental diseases by shock methods has attracted widespread attention, and because it is utilized in practically every large mental institution, the techniques are a vital part of every course in modern psychiatric training.

The insulin shock treatment has been exceptionally useful in the treatment of the schizophrenic psychoses, particularly in those patients who have not been ill more than six or eight months. European clinics report as high as 75 per cent recoveries in such acute cases and in this country, where the evaluation of this treatment is more conservative, the recovery rate is conceded to be definitely higher than it was before the insulin shock therapy was employed.

Metrazol and electric shock treatment produce results almost as good as those secured by insulin, particularly in the catatonic forms. Metrazol, however, is more useful in the treatment of involutional melancholia and other depressed states, but because of the tendency of dislocations of the shoulders and hip, and because compression fractures of the vertebrae are so frequent, much doubt has arisen as to the advisability of its use. Because of these undesirable side actions the metrazol treatment has been replaced by electric shock in most institutions.

Insulin Routine

Insulin shock therapy was introduced into psychiatry in 1933 by Manfred Sakel who first used insulin in treating drug addicts. From his observations of these patients he was encouraged to use large doses of insulin in the excited mental states, particularly schizophrenia.

The Insulin Schedule.—The method consists essentially of the induction of a series of severe hypoglycemic shocks. Therapy starts with a small dose of insulin, about 15 to 20 units, and the dose is increased daily by about 10 units until hypoglycemic shock is produced. When the required dose has been ascertained, a series of severe shocks is induced. The number of shocks induced varies greatly with the mental condition of the patient. In general, 20 to 40 shocks are given; however, this may be increased to as many as 80 or even 100. Some authorities feel that insulin therapy should not be discontinued as valueless until the patient has had 40 hypoglycemic shocks.

Therapy is administered every day except for one or two days a week, the so-called rest days when no treatment is given. The insulin is usually given in the morning on a fasting stomach.

The Insulin Coma.—During the first one or two hours after the insulin injection, the patient becomes progressively more somnolent and has profuse perspiration. The somnolence may be interrupted at times by excitement, which is usually transitory. Usually about three or four hours after the injection of insulin the somnolence gradually terminates in coma. Insulin coma varies considerably in depth, depending on the dose of insulin, the duration of the coma, and the patient's ability to mobilize glucose from his own glycogen stores. In light coma the patient may be partially aroused although he is unable to make contact with his environment. At this stage all the reflexes are intact, and there are no pathologic reflexes. As the coma deepens, the tendon reflexes decrease in activity and pathological reflexes appear, such as the

Babinski and Hoffmann signs. In very deep coma all the reflexes disappear, and the muscles are atonic. During the course of insulin coma the pulse usually becomes slow unless excitement intervenes. It may even go below 40. The temperature may fall as low as 30° C. During the coma the patient may have sporadic muscle twitchings, but usually no epileptic seizure occurs. The above described reaction is the usual type and is sometimes referred to as a "wet shock."

Occasionally a patient does not show a great deal of somnolence and perspiration after receiving insulin, but in the second or third hour he may suddenly have an epileptic seizure. This reaction is sometimes termed a "dry shock" in contradistinction to wet shock. Dry shock is not very frequent as compared with wet shock.

The number of periods of coma and the duration and depth of coma vary a great deal and depend upon the judgment of the physician. In general, paranoid patients and patients with catatonic excitement are allowed to have periods of coma lasting one to three hours, or sometimes even longer; whereas, the patients who are in catatonic stupor are brought out of hypoglycemic shock when they are excited.

Epileptic seizures are sometimes used for therapeutic purposes during hypoglycemic shock. Sometimes these are actually induced by giving the patient metrazol while he is in hypoglycemic shock. However, after an epileptic seizure the patient should be taken out of shock. After an epileptic seizure the patient usually comes out of shock spontaneously, but, if he is not given carbohydrates, he may relapse into hypoglycemia.

Nursing Care.—Insulin is given on a fasting stomach usually in the morning. After administration of the insulin the patient is put to bed and remains under the supervision of a nurse until treatment is concluded and the patient is fully conscious. Several patients may be treated together in a ward. The pulse is checked at frequent intervals. The patient's color is noted and also the type of respiration. The following materials should be available for immediate use:

1 Sterile 50 c.c. syringe (large sterile syringes for intravenous injection of glucose).

1 Sterile 2 c.c. syringe (small sterile syringes for injection of adrenalin, etc.).

Sterile needles for intravenous injection.

Sterile 50 per cent glucose solution.

Ampoules of adrenalin, caffeine, and coramin.

Glucose solution for administration through nasal tube; a 30 per cent glucose solution is most convenient.

Alcohol, iodine, and sponges.

Rubber tourniquet.

Nasal tube.

A lubricant such as glycerin for the nasal tube.

A syringe to aspirate the nasal tube to ascertain if it is in the stomach.

Mouth gags.

Termination of Coma.—Hypoglycemic coma is usually terminated by administering glucose, or another sugar solution, through a nasal tube. The nasal tube may be introduced at the beginning of the coma as a precaution and kept in place with a few strips of adhesive until it has to be used. Before using the tube, the nurse should make certain that it is in the stomach, by aspirating gastric juice with a syringe. If no gastric juice is obtained, a quick push on the plunger produces a characteristic rumbling which seems to come from the

50 Treatments of Insulin -
pulse below 40 & above 120 -
cheyne stokes resp.

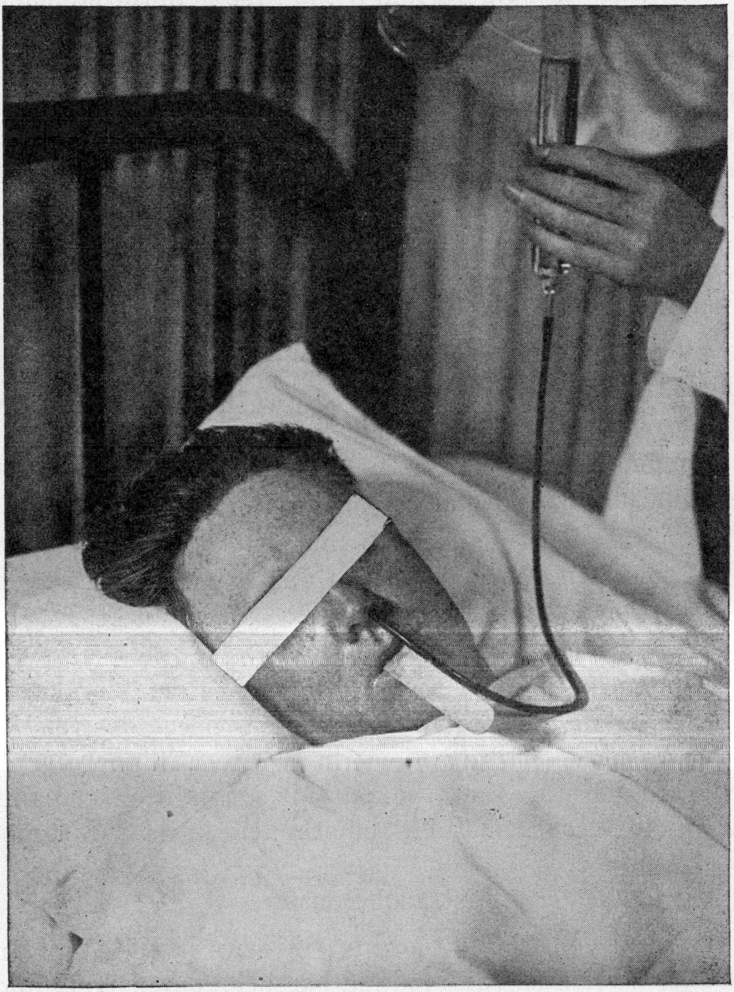

Fig. 35.—A patient in insulin shock. The nasal tube has been previously introduced and the technique is shown for terminating the coma with glucose solution. The tongue blade is in place to protect the tongue and lips from injury during convulsive twitching of the jaw.

1.5 Gm Glucose.
for q Unit of Insulin,

epigastrium and a vibration that can usually be felt by the hand on the epigastrium if the tube is in the stomach. The patient usually regains consciousness 15 to 30 minutes after receiving glucose through the nasal tube. If an emergency arises, 50 per cent glucose can be given intravenously. Patients respond almost immediately to intravenous glucose. Adrenalin intramuscularly will also quickly alleviate hypoglycemic coma but is rarely used unless in an emergency a vein cannot be found in which to inject the glucose.

After the patient has recovered consciousness, he may be allowed to get up. A meal should always be given soon after recovering consciousness, or else the patient may go back into a state of shock.

Danger Signs.—The indications for the immediate termination of shock are:

1. Irregular pulse or rate under 40 per minute.
2. Sudden, marked fluctuations in pulse.
3. Cheyne-Stokes respirations.
4. Marked cyanosis of the face.

If the nurse observes any of the above signs, she should immediately notify the physician. It is necessary for the nurse to be constantly alert during insulin therapy in order to be sure that the patient's condition remains satisfactory, as sometimes emergencies arise at a moment's notice.

Metrazol Routine

Metrazol convulsive therapy since its introduction in 1935 by Ladislaus von Meduna has been extensively and widely used. At first it was restricted to the treatment of schizophrenia, but later its application was extended to other psychoses, especially manic-depressive psychoses and involutional melancholia, and even the neuroses.

The Nature of Metrazol.—Clinically metrazol is penta-methylene-tetrazol. It was synthesized by Schmidt of Heidelberg in an effort to obtain water soluble substances having the therapeutic properties of camphor.

Metrazol is a stimulant. In doses of 0.1 to 0.2 gram it stimulates respiration and circulation by its action on the medullary nuclei. In larger doses it is a convulsant. In a 10 per cent solution it can be injected subcutaneously, intramuscularly, or intravenously. When administered intravenously, it disappears rapidly from the circulation, so that it must be injected quickly to produce a convulsion. It is very easily antagonized by sedatives. Sedatives administered the night before will often prevent a metrazol convulsion.

Contraindications.—Patients are given a thorough physical examination before being given metrazol therapy. Each patient has a blood sugar and blood urea nitrogen determination as well as a urinalysis to make sure the blood and urinary constituents are normal. The contraindications are:

1. Any acute febrile condition.
2. Decompensating cardiovascular disease.
3. Marked and persistent hypertension.
4. Severe anemia.
5. Any abnormality in blood chemistry.
6. History of previous severe head injury with subsequent unconsciousness.
7. Poorly calcified bones.

Metrazol treatments are omitted during the menstrual periods.

The Metrazol Schedule.—Patients are given a metrazol treatment three times a week on alternate days. It is administered in the morning with the patient fasting.

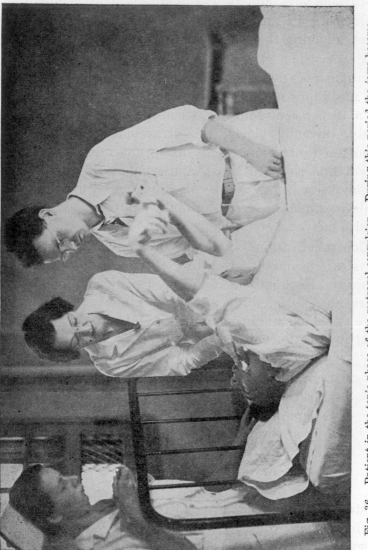

Fig. 36.—Patient in the tonic phase of the metrazol convulsion. During this period the jaws become widely separated and a gauze or rubber gag is introduced to protect the tongue from being bitten.

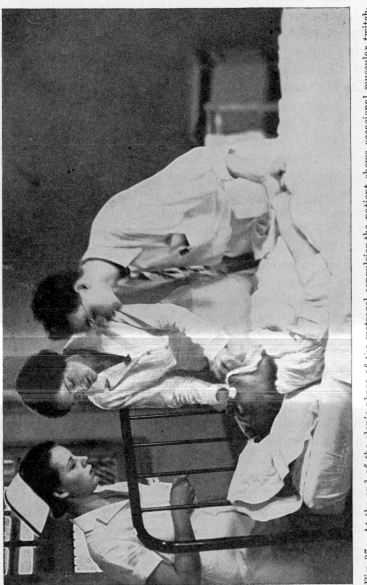

Fig. 37.—At the end of the clonic phase of the metrazol convulsion the patient shows occasional muscular twitching; the skin is slightly cyanotic and normal respiration is about to begin.

The temperature, pulse, respiration, and blood pressure are taken twice daily. The initial dose is 0.4 or 0.5 gram intravenously in a 10 per cent aqueous solution. Usually during the course of therapy the convulsive threshold rises, necessitating an increase in dosage.

The Metrazol Convulsion.—The convulsion usually begins ten or fifteen seconds after the injection. Occasionally it may be delayed for a minute or two. A few seconds before the convulsion, the patient frequently becomes restless, bewildered, apprehensive, or even terrified and usually coughs once or twice. The convulsion begins with a few rapid clonic twitches of the facial muscles and the upper extremities which quickly give way to a tonic contraction involving the entire musculature. The fingers are flexed, the upper and lower extremities extended with the feet in plantar flexion and the body in opisthotonos. At the onset of the tonic contraction, the mouth is opened wide for a few seconds. The tonic phase lasts ten to twenty seconds and is succeeded by the clonic phase, the tonic contractions being interrupted by short periods of relaxation which gradually lengthen until a typical clonic convulsion is present. The clonic contractions gradually decrease in frequency and usually stop in fifteen to forty seconds, leaving the patient cyanotic and apneic. Stertorous respirations then begin and the cyanosis disappears. Occasionally respirations are delayed a few seconds, but tapping the chest or one or two attempts at artificial respiration instantly initiates them.

Consciousness gradually returns five or ten minutes after the convulsion. On awakening, the patient is confused and dazed and frequently thrashes about in bed aimlessly, or attempts to get up. In most cases this period of confusion is followed by a sleep of one-half to two hours' duration. On awakening, the patient has amnesia for the convulsion. Sometimes he recalls the anxiety following the injection and sometimes recalls aurae such as flashes of light, dizziness, or tinnitus.

Nursing Care.—The patient is placed flat in bed and is dressed in a loosely fitting gown. The bed should be far enough away from the walls and other obstacles so that the patient cannot strike his limbs against them during a convulsion. The following materials should be provided on a cart or tray so that they may be carried from patient to patient:

Sterile 10-20 c.c. syringes.
Sterile needles.
Metrazol in 30 or 100 c.c. rubber-stoppered bottles.
Respiratory and circulatory stimulants ready for immediate use, such as alpha lobeline, epinephrine, caffeine sodiobenzoate, and sodium amytal, or other anticonvulsants which can be given intravenously.
Tourniquet.
Arm board.
Alcohol sponges.
Dry sponges.
Tincture of iodine or some other antiseptic.
Mouth gags.

The needles used should be of sufficiently large bore so that the metrazol can be injected quickly. The mouth gags can be made of cellucotton rolled tightly with gauze bandage. They are about four inches long and three-quarters of an inch in diameter.

A nurse assists the physician, going from patient to patient with him, handing him the syringe and other articles as required. Considerable time can be saved if the nurse fills the syringes with the prescribed dosage of metrazol before therapy is started. The syringes can then be laid in the order in which they will be used. The nurse has a chart on which is recorded the patient's temperature, pulse, respiration, and blood pressure of that morning, the present and previous dose of metrazol, and the type of reaction the patient had at his last treatment. The nurse records the time in seconds from the injection to the appearance of the convulsion and also the duration of the convulsion.

A second nurse prepares the arm for injection. Several attendants should be present to hold the patient if he resists the injection. The mouth gag is inserted at the beginning of the convulsion. Usually the mouth is opened wide at the start of the convulsion, providing ample opportunity to insert the gag.

After the convulsion the respiration and pulse are recorded. The doctor and assistant nurse remain with the patient until his condition is satisfactory, as manifested by regular pulse and respiration and the disappearance of cyanosis. A nurse is assigned to remain with the patient to see that his condition remains satisfactory and that he does not injure himself, for not infrequently for five or ten minutes after the convulsion the patient is confused and restless and may toss and roll about the bed. This period of restlessness is usually followed by sleep lasting one-half to two hours. After the patients are asleep, it is necessary to have only one nurse watch several patients. On awakening, the patient sometimes complains of nausea and headache, but usually he may be allowed up and given a regular diet.

The nurse on metrazol wards should be alert and report any aches or pains that the patients may complain of, as fractures, particularly of the vertebrae, may occur during a convulsion. Since many of the patients do not like and even dread the treatment, the nurse should use every opportunity to allay their fears and reassure them about the therapy.

Complications.—Dislocation of the jaw occurs not infrequently. This is manifested immediately after the convulsion by the patient's inability to close his mouth. The lower jaw is depressed and protrudes so that the lower teeth are anterior to the upper teeth. Occasionally the humerus is dislocated. Sometimes fractures occur; the most frequent is a compression fracture of the vertebrae, usually the thoracic vertebrae, but fractures of other bones, such as the humerus and even the femur, may occur.

Electric Shock Therapy

Electrical shock is by far the most convenient and practical form of shock therapy. Introduced in 1938 by Cerletti and Bini, two Italian clinicians, after ample experimentation on dogs, it is now being used with good results in the depressions, particularly involutional melancholia. To less extent, it has been valuable in the catatonic form of schizophrenia, in mania, and in certain psychoneuroses.

Contraindications.—These are the same as for any convulsant therapy and include such conditions as hypertensive cardiorenal disease, active tuberculosis, acute infections and severe debility. Electric shock can be given to elderly patients even up to 70 years, with greater safety than one can apply metrazol or insulin therapy. Fractures are far less common than in the metrazol treatment.

Advantages.—By far the greatest advantages electric shock possesses over all other types of treatment is the simplicity of the procedure. Moreover, it is decidedly easier on the patient. The extreme fear of successive treatments which has made metrazol objectionable does not occur in electric shock, because the patient is rendered unconscious immediately, and there is no memory of the shock. After a treatment, the patient usually lies quietly, does not become terrorized and remains receptive to further treatment. Electric shock treatments do not produce as harmful an effect on the heart and blood vessels as does metrazol.

The Electric Shock Schedule.—Treatments are usually given two or three times a week, in the morning, on a fasting stomach.

Nursing Care.—The nurse in charge should prepare the following materials on a tray which is placed conveniently near the treatment table:

Respiratory stimulants (a) Metrazol (b) Coramine.

Airway tube, tongue retractor and mouth gag.

Syringe with hypodermic and intravenous needles.

A jar of electrode jelly.

One quart of 20% saline solution for soaking the electrodes.

The patient is placed on a padded wooden table with a hard pillow under the dorsal spine to prevent fractures of the vertebrae. All metal articles such as hair pins and artificial dentures are removed from the patient's person.

Electrode jelly containing pumice stone is applied liberally to each side of the head in the fronto-parietal region.

After the convulsion, the respiration and pulse are recorded. At the same time, all data as to voltage, duration of current and other pertinent items should be obtained from the physician and entered on the patient's chart. The patient should be carefully watched because for a variable time, he may be very restless, may fumble with the bed clothes, try to get up or may drop off into a deep sleep. Recovery is usually complete in ten to thirty minutes.

The Apparatus.—The machine is a fairly simple electric device consisting of a stimulating unit and a pair of metal electrodes which are fixed to a chrome metal frame very much resembling a pair of obstetrical forceps. In some models the electrodes are set upon a simple metal

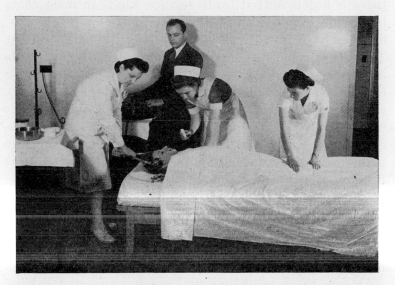

Fig. 38.—A demonstration of the technique of electrical shock. The head clamps are in position, the mouth gag is poised for use, the knees are held firmly in the relaxed position, and the current is about to be applied.

head band. The machine is equipped with two circuits, one for measuring the patient's head resistance and the other which is connected to the electrodes and which delivers an A.C. current with a maximum voltage of 140. Automatically, the duration of the current through the head is limited to $\frac{1}{10}$ to .15 seconds. The electrodes are covered with a piece of linen and are then soaked in

20 per cent salt solution. After measuring the patient's head resistance, the switch is changed to the treatment circuit, the voltmeter set at the agreed voltage, usually 70 volts, and the time stop switch set at .1 second.

The Convulsion.—Before the shock is administered, a gauze roll is placed between the patient's teeth. When the current is applied, the patient immediately loses consciousness lasting for a few seconds. During this period, there is a generalized tonic seizure which in most cases is strong enough to cause the patient to clamp the jaws, flex the head and trunk and assume a sitting posture. The face is usually flushed, but later pales, the pulse rate is increased, blood pressure rises rapidly and the pupils may become widely dilated. As consciousness returns, the patient is confused, talks incoherently and is unable to recall anything about the treatment. All this, however, disappears in a few minutes although a certain proportion of the patients will demonstrate an amnesia for several days after the treatment.

If the initial tonic seizure is followed by clonic spasms, the face and lips show considerable cyanosis, and there is frothing at the mouth. The seizure is a typical grand mal and resembles in many respects the reaction to metrazol.

During the convulsion, the jaw is supported to prevent dislocation. The arms are held to the sides of the chest, and the knees are held together, but convulsive movements must not be restricted so as to prevent fractures and dislocations.

Results.—In the treatment of depressions, particularly involutional melancholia, improvement begins early and is usually noted after the first two or three seizures. Recovery occurs after a series of only six to ten convulsive shocks. Treatment is discontinued when the patient attains a state of well-being, is no longer morbid and is free of agitation. If symptoms reappear, a second series of treatments is given. As with any other form of shock treatment, when the patient's emotional tone improves, an excellent opportunity is provided for airing out the psychic stresses which have contributed to the mental upset.

References

Jessner, Lucie and Ryan, V. Gerard: Shock Treatment in Psychiatry: A Manual, New York, 1941, Grune and Stratton, Inc.

Noyes, Arthur: Modern Clinical Psychiatry, ed. 2, Philadelphia, 1939, W. B. Saunders Co.

Sakel, Manfred: Pharmacological Shock Treatment of Schizophrenia, New York, 1937, Nervous and Mental Disease Publishing Co.

Questions for Chapter XXVII

Shock Therapy

1. For what psychosis is insulin shock most beneficial?
2. Describe the manifestations of an insulin coma. Differentiate between "wet" and "dry" shock.
3. What materials should be available for emergency use in the shock routine?
4. What danger signs indicate an immediate termination of insulin shock?
5. Who introduced metrazol shock therapy? What is the physiological action of this drug?
6. What sedatives must be avoided when this treatment is proposed? Describe a typical metrazol convulsion.
7. What articles would you have prepared on the tray for this treatment?
8. Discuss complications which might arise during metrazol therapy.
9. Describe the after-care of patients who have just received the metrazol treatment.
10. What are the two outstanding advantages of electric shock therapy as compared with metrazol?
11. How was this form of shock treatment introduced?
12. In preparation for a treatment, what articles are necessary as a part of the technique?
13. Describe the procedure and the instrument which is used in electric shock treatment.
14. In what conditions is this treatment particularly beneficial?

CHAPTER XXVIII

PSYCHIATRY AND THE LAW

Neither physician nor nurse should be utterly ignorant of the rudimentary principles of law which concern themselves with the mental patient and his legal status. A psychiatric nurse should be sufficiently acquainted with the legal aspects of psychiatry to spare her from various embarrassing and distressing predicaments in which she may innocently and unwittingly find herself.

The legal significance of psychiatry is of special concern because mental disease affects the behavior of the individual and his reaction to others. Where behavior varies considerably from those standards laid down by society, the person is considered either a criminal or insane. It should be emphasized that the term insanity is a legal one and not medical. According to Singer and Krohn, the *definition for legal insanity* is as follows: "An insane person or lunatic is one in whom there exists, due to disease, a more or less prolonged deviation from his normal method of behavior and who is, therefore, incapable of managing his affairs or transacting ordinary business, who is dangerous to himself, to others, or to property, or who interferes with the peace of society." The definition does not include the idiot or imbecile. The determination of insanity in a legal sense is based upon the particular act or misbehavior in each case, and each case must therefore be tried on its own merits.

If an individual is guilty of a crime by reason of insanity, he is committed to an institution not so much to protect society as to receive the benefits of treatment. This is a step in a more humane and rational direction, for it implies that the wrongdoer is not a criminal but is mentally ill.

Every state has made some sort of provision for the care and treatment of the mentally ill. In most instances this consists of a state hospital system consisting of one or more institutions. In a few states the actual care is left in the hands of county authorities, but under a close inspection by state officials.

Methods of Commitment.—There is no uniformity of commitment methods in the several states, but no one can be deprived of his liberty without due process of law. In a few parts of this country the commitment proceedings still imply that the mentally ill person is a criminal in that he must be tried by jury. A jury is not always competent to decide on such delicate and technical matters as to whether or not a person has a mental ailment, and the entire ordeal is such that it may often act as a great psychological shock to the patient.

It is much better to simplify the legal side of commitment and to reduce it to a simple and very informal procedure but at the same time protecting the individual's legal and constitutional rights. In general the commitment proceedings consist of three parts, (a) the application, (b) the examination, and (c) the detention in some type of institution.

The action is initiated generally by relatives or friends who have become aware of the mental abnormality. Any legally appointed officer of the law, a policeman, a sheriff or his deputies, members of charitable organizations, a public health official, or any private citizen may make the application which will bring the matter to the attention of the proper court. In most states the court which functions in settling matters of insanity is the common pleas court or the probate court. Here the application is submitted; statements by interested parties are heard under oath; and all available information about the patient and his behavior is recorded.

Frequently the application must be accompanied by the certificates of one or more physicians. The judge may, however, appoint one or two physicians to conduct the psychiatric examination. Specially certified physicians who make medicolegal examinations and submit their opinions to the court are known as alienists. Each alienist must satisfy himself that mental disease exists before he can lawfully certify the patient for commitment. The testimony of lay witnesses and of the examining physicians must be sufficient to convince a judge or jury that the person in question is a social menace and needs to be restrained and treated.

If the court finds that the need exists for institutionalization, the patient is generally committed to a state hospital. In some localities provision is made for temporary commitment in a detention hospital. This observation period is usually from five to thirty days, and during this interval additional data are obtained to determine whether or not final action is justified.

Legal Rights of the Confined Mental Patient.—Every nurse who has charge of mental patients in an institution should be acquainted with the legal status of such patients. Statutes provide for certain rights, even though the patient be already certified as insane. A patient may be allowed to have visitors, may send unopened letters to judges and hospital staff members, and may make contact with attorneys. However, both nurse and doctor may exercise a reasonable control over the matter of the patient's correspondence. If by reason of his psychosis a patient is dangerously paranoid or maniacal and may take to writing threatening, abusive, or obscene letters to strangers or public officials, it is better to distract the individual by encouraging other activities or to turn over such missives to relatives, who can dispose of them without causing undue concern or worry to others.

Many people still believe that a goodly number of patients are confined in mental hospitals without good reason or justification. Actually, under the present methods of commitment such a miscarriage of justice is rare or next to impossible. Where illegal detention is suspected any individual is free to force court action through *habeas corpus* proceedings. By this means the patient can be brought to court for a hearing and the cause for confinement must be clearly shown by those who detain him.

Patients in state hospitals cannot, under ordinary circumstances, be treated by their own personal physicians, and neither do the latter usually care to assume such responsibilities. The directing head of the hospital usually decides the question of medical consultation but may, as a matter of pure courtesy, allow the family physician to visit the patient.

A patient who has been adjudicated as insane loses his right to citizenship, and this cannot be regained until such time as he recovers full mental capacity. Neither can a certified patient enter into a valid contract unless it can be proved that such contract was made during a lucid interval. Even the simple endorsement of a check can be regarded as illegal if the patient has been committed and confined for mental disease.

Guardianship.—To protect the patient's rights and property, a guardian is appointed either by the court which commits him or by the state authorities. If the amount of property warrants the expense of guardianship or if necessary business involving such property is transacted, the guardian's responsibilities are n o t trivial. In some states this property guardian is called a conservator. A guardian of the person of the patient is one who has direct responsibility for the patient's personal welfare. He is generally a near relative. He cannot confine the patient in an institution without permission or approval of the court but can dictate, within certain limits, the nature of the patient's treatment, and he can sign a permit for a major operation. He may also have custody of the minor children of the patient if the mother is incapable of this herself.

The wife or husband of a patient, rather than the parents, is regarded as the natural guardian. Every guardian must give bond for the proper performance of his duties. At regular intervals he is required to make an accounting of expenses and income. His first consideration must be the comfort of the patient; he must not be so penurious as to favor the interests of the family at the expense of the patient's welfare.

Parole and Discharge.—In most states at the discretion of the directing physician, patients may be permitted to return to their homes on parole for a period of a few days, a few weeks, or even a year. This parole is a "trying-out" period during which the patient can demonstrate the degree of recovery as measured by his capacity to readjust himself to normal social conditions. The patient, however, remains under the supervision of the hospital and must continue to submit to regular mental examinations. If the parole record is satisfactory, the patient may then be legally discharged.

Usually the legal discharge of a mental patient is not as formal a procedure as is the commitment. The hospital physicians in a staff meeting make a final examination, and the superintendent merely issues the order for release. The patient may be discharged because he has recovered or is greatly improved or because his relatives have made satisfactory arrangements for treatment in a private institution. This does not, however, apply to the patient who is criminally insane, as he is subject to the orders of a regular criminal court.

In all instances in which a patient has been legally discharged, the hospital authorities notify the court which has been responsible for the commitment, to this effect.

Voluntary Commitment.—The most desirable manner of obtaining treatment for mental disease is voluntary commitment. Unfortunately this is not frequently done because, in most mental afflictions, insight into one's own mental condition is poor, and the average patient will not of his own volition go to a hospital. Under voluntary commitment the patient need not go through any humiliating court action, but simply signs an application and agrees to submit himself for treatment and to abide by the rules of the hospital. By doing this, he will neither lose his rights as a citizen nor commit himself for an indefinite period. Upon giving three days' notice he is entitled to leave the hospital. If in the judgment of the physician in charge, however, his being discharged constitutes a menace to the community, relatives can be quickly notified, a legal commitment can be arranged and further detention assured. Otherwise the patient under voluntary commitment is free to go, with no other formality.

Mental Capacity in Making a Will.—The question as to the mental capacity of elderly people making a will, i.e., the testamentary capacity, is often an important problem in legal psychiatry. A nurse who is in charge of an aging patient may frequently be called upon for testimony as to his testamentary capacity; she may be asked to witness the signature to a will or even to draw up a will. It is rather important for her to have in mind the important considerations necessary to establish or to recognize whether or not a patient can make or sign a will.

As a rule, a patient who is able to carry on his ordinary business is qualified. Where, however, an individual has been an invalid for some length of time and has not clearly demonstrated this capacity, it should be ascertained whether he has an understanding and knowledge of his business or vocation, whether his memory is such that he knows what property he possesses, whether he has a knowledge of the persons or organizations to whom he desires to will his property, and whether he shows reasonably good judgment pertaining to the disposal of his property.

Senile individuals may have periods of mental clouding and confusion, but they may also have lucid intervals. A will is legal if it is made during a lucid period as long as it can be proved that such a period of mental clarity existed at the time.

The question of testamentary capacity in the mental patient, particularly in the old person, is always a trying one, as indicated by the frequent legal controversies which arise between beneficiaries and nonbeneficiaries when considerable property is involved.

Privileged Communications.—This is a legal term which refers to any matter or information held in necessary professional confidence as between a patient and a physician which is not admissible as evidence in a court. It is an evasion of the law to submit in evidence on the witness stand any facts dealing with methods of treatment. The psychiatric nurse should, therefore, be reminded that the medical chart and the data thereon can be regarded as privileged communication. It is a part of her duty to protect this record from scrutiny by unauthorized or curious individuals. If any doubt arises as to rights and privileges in this respect, the matter should be referred to the administrative officers of the hospital or to the physician in charge.

References

Singer and Krohn: Insanity and Law, Philadelphia, 1924, P. Blakiston's Son & Co.

Sullivan, W. C.: Crime and Insanity, New York, 1925, Physicians and Surgeons Book Co.

White, William Allen: Crimes and Criminals, New York, 1933, Farrar and Rinehart.

Questions for Chapter XXVIII
Psychiatry and the Law

1. Why must legal procedures be followed in committing a mental patient to an institution?
2. What is meant by "legal insanity"?
3. Discuss the methods of commitment to a mental hospital. What are the specific regulations in your state?
4. Who may apply for the commitment of a mentally ill patient? Where would he apply for it?
5. What are the legal rights of a confined mental patient?
6. Could a patient legally adjudged insane vote by proxy, inherit money, or sign checks?
7. What provision can be made to legalize the patient's business affairs?
8. Discuss parole and discharge of mentally ill patients.
9. Is voluntary commitment possible?
10. What is meant by the term "testamentary capacity"? What is the nurse's duty if asked to witness a will?
11. Why is the mentally ill patient's chart considered "privileged communication"? Can anyone have access to this chart? What do you understand this term to mean?

CHAPTER XXIX
MENTAL HYGIENE

Psychiatry has rapidly developed into a body of knowledge which has found useful application in many fields. It has contributed its share in bringing forth some understanding of mind, of human emotions, and of their interactions in personal and social life. Through the application of all the social sciences, man is beginning to appreciate some of his childish attitudes and his senseless cravings which disrupt his health and happiness—individually and socially.

Mental hygiene is a concerted movement or plan which gathers what knowledge and means are at hand and proposes to seek out the sources of mental havoc, to do everything possible to offset these influences, to promote the development of the best mental conditions in everyone, and so far as possible, to correct mental disorder as it now exists by fostering research and promoting adequate psychiatric and institutional care.

No program could be more courageous and comprehensive. It implies the cooperation of every social force which promotes the betterment of man as an individual and as a member of the social group. Mental hygiene is a meeting ground of all the social sciences. At the very inception of the mental hygiene movement in 1908 it demonstrated its breadth of vision when it invited to its first formal meeting a judge, a lawyer, a minister, a psychiatrist, a general practitioner, a hospital manager, several members of the faculty of a university, and the members of a family of one who had been a mental patient.

Hygienic efforts to control mental disease are naturally matters of prevention. Because the sources of mental disease are manifold and because many of the causes still remain a deep mystery, one can readily appreciate the immensity of the task which mental hygiene has assigned itself.

Fundamental aims of the program are the following preventive measures:

a. To apply what knowledge of human heredity is available so as to prevent the birth of the mentally useless.

b. To promote good physical health during growth and development.

c. To improve working conditions and economic conditions which would eliminate overwork and undernourishment.

d. To promote natural and healthy emotional attitudes in the family circle and in the social relationships of the community.

e. To encourage sound methods of education and training, particularly of children, so that personality is given every opportunity for normal development and natural elementary habits and attitudes are established.

Child Guidance.—Most of the progress in mental hygiene in the past two decades has been in the field of child guidance. This activity has attained great importance, and it now includes the study of the problems of mental and physical growth, of deliquency, dependency, child welfare, and child placement. Physicians who are specially trained in the field of child guidance are known as orthopsychiatrists.

"It is because the child is plastic," says Dr. William A. White, "and is capable within limitations of being molded by circumstances, that childhood is the most im-

child guidance - studies first normal child - then abnormal - behavior of child.

portant period of life and the golden period for mental hygiene.'' The study of the child's responses to his environment gives the clues to the trends, both good and bad, of the personality in later years. Between the ages of 2 and 6 years, while the child is still completely under the influence of its home environment, most of the habit patterns and attitudes toward the environment which are to determine the emotional characteristics of the adult person are set down.

The growing child is a far more complex phenomenon than the adult in that he is constantly changing in the total structure of his personality and in his individual traits, while the grown person settles into a more constant and ''set'' pattern. Hence several divergent approaches must be used to arrive at a complete understanding of the child and his behavior. The orthopsychiatrist must draw on various fields to complete his knowledge—he must be familiar with sociology and psychology; he must know the physical as well as the psychiatric components in his little patient before he can arrive at any useful conclusions.

The social factors which leave their imprint on the child's personality can never be slighted. Exposure of children to gross neglect and extreme poverty, alcoholism in the parents, broken homes, illegitimacy, and mental deficiency are examples. Perhaps equally potent in disturbing the emotional atmosphere of the home are temperamental differences, disagreements over religious beliefs, frequent changes in residence, and lack of normal recreation and outside interests.

The psychological considerations in understanding the growing child are chiefly those which deal with mental development. The intellectual growth of the child should be carefully checked by periodic mental measurements,

M. Hygiene — System of living whereby
person achieves optinum of
happiness & effeciency

MENTAL HYGIENE   317

for some of the emotional problems of childhood can be
caused by the strain of a mentally backward individual
attempting to keep up with his more normal brothers
and sisters. The precocious or bright child may be a
problem because his special capabilities are not recognized and directed into useful and healthful channels
and find expression in bad habits and mischievous behavior. A psychological study should also include an
investigation of special disabilities such as are associated
with abnormal handedness or which are manifested by
speech disorders, stammering, stuttering, etc.

The third consideration in child guidance is the physical status. A complete physical examination is necessary to rule out disease which may be a serious handicap to personality development. Focal infection, enlarged tonsils and adenoids, and deficiency disease due to
faulty diet are frequent causes of poor mental health.
Some physicians overemphasize the influence of the endocrine glands in the causation of nervous disorders and
abnormal personality traits. It is probably true that
some children with gross deviation in physical development have a serious glandular defect. Many such disorders can be adequately treated by proper glandular
replacement therapy.

Finally the psychiatric approach is necessary to understand the child in his entirety. In this general analysis the physician can usually reveal the keystone of
misbehavior. Only a few examples of some of the faulty
elementary habits and attitudes which a psychiatric
study will often disclose can be cited in this discussion.

a. Bad eating habits. Finickiness and unreasonable-
ness about food. It is usually revealed that these attitudes are often used as a means of gaining some special
advantage. Child Problems -

Irritability   —   truancy —   Backwardness
  Jealousy —   Destructiveness   Shyness in school
Temper tantrum —   feeding problems —   Fears —
Delinquency .   Thumbsucking —
Stealing   Nailbiting ;
Sex misdemeanors   Dishonesty

b. Irregular sleep habits. A wrong understanding of dreams.

c. Wrong attitudes toward play. A spirit of poor sportsmanship. Exaggerated aggressiveness or recessiveness with others.

d. Abnormally implanted fears and frights.

e. Faulty utilization of the emotions such as rage, disgust, abnormal likes and dislikes.

f. Excessive attachment to other members of the family.

g. Distorted conception of sexual matters.

h. A sense of physical inferiority because of some deformity or pronounced physical characteristic.

i. Too much ado about minor illness and overemphasis on simple bodily complaints.

j. Poor reaction to the competitive atmosphere of the schoolroom.

To lay out a constructive program in child guidance compels the physician to seek the cooperation of every person and every agency which deals with the child. This means a most intimate coordination of interests on the part of parents, teachers, social workers, and visiting nurses. Teachers should be trained in the early recognition and detection of these problems. Since a large number of cases of abnormal behavior are brought to light for the first time in the school, a child guidance clinic in conjunction with the school system is a decided advantage.

Nervousness in children is based on a tangible organic disturbance in less than 25 per cent of all cases. By far the vast majority of personality disorders in children belong to the so-called reactive-behavior group, meaning that the trouble is essentially in the emotional life of the young person. Examples of this are temper tan-

Fundamentally our difficulties are no different than others —
Regard mental poise + adaptability as Keyboard to
MENTAL HYGIENE *good mental* 319 *health —*

trums, habitual lying, stealing, excessive timidity, masturbation, and general delinquency. True mental disease is exceedingly rare.

Mental Hygiene in Adolescence.—Adolescence is a period of great instability and is generally associated with increased self-consciousness and frequently with an overwhelming sense of inferiority. At the same time there is an enormous increase in psychic and physical energy which demands expression through several main trends of activity. The adolescent discovers new powers and new capacities to accomplish tasks in his own way. He becomes self-assertive in religious, social, and vocational activities; he manifests a desire not only to emulate, but to improve upon, the accomplishments of his elders. Instinctual energies are directed away from family attachments. There is a gradual emancipation from emotional dependence on the parents. Friendships with individuals of the same sex outside the home are established. Contact with the opposite sex in a natural and easy manner indicates the normal development of heterosexual instincts and the gradual ripening into adulthood.

This great period of transition from childhood to maturity is fraught with great dangers if the understructure of a normal, healthy childhood is lacking, if a sound moral training has been overlooked or if there develop at this time certain arrests of growth, particularly in the psychosexual spheres. Out of the adolescent years emerge the unstable personalities, the petty offender, the psychopath, and the young criminal. It is an established fact that most criminal careers begin between the ages of fifteen and twenty-five. The instinct for acquisition is prominent and the restless craving for adventure and excitement is frequently directed through bad associations into dangerous antisocial channels. Equally distressing is the arrest of personality at this age which

Use suggestions & learn how to use surroundings as to your success of happiness.

expresses itself in poor social and heterosexual adjustment and compels the young person to retreat into the shell of his inner life—there to live in a world of his own construction away from a life of usefulness and successful adaptation. In this introverted adolescent personality one sees the tragic mental disasters which the psychiatrist recognizes as schizophrenia.

Mental hygiene proposes to recognize these pernicious trends and encourages every endeavor to place the individual, with due regard for his inherent capacities, into that setting where he may have the greatest potentialities for a happy and successful adjustment to the demands of life.

Mental Hygiene in the Community.—The more that more people know about the forces which act upon the human mind to produce mental disease, the sooner shall be consummated those ideals set down by the mental hygiene campaign. The dissemination of this knowledge can only be a slow and painstaking process. Parent education, public lectures, periodicals, books written in popular vein, and other methods of publicizing information on mental health are proving invaluable in promoting the cause of mental hygiene. The public health nurse with psychiatric training, because of her intimate contact with the home life of her patients and her immediate knowledge of the social and economic factors which affect her charges, can function as a most useful teacher and worker in the field of mental hygiene.

References

Adamson, Elizabeth I.: So You're Going to a Psychiatrist, New York, 1936, Thomas Y. Crowell Company.

Anderson, Camilla M.: Emotional Hygiene, New York, 1937, J. B. Lippincott Co.

Campbell, Charles M.: Human Personality and the Environment, New York, 1934, The Macmillan Company.

I Q = Mental Age over Chronological Age
autistic thinking = Daydreaming, or preoccupied.
schizophrenic and manic preoccupied.
MENTAL HYGIENE   321

Eyre, Mary B.: Psychology and Mental Hygiene for Nurses, New York, 1922, The Macmillan Company.

Gesell, Arnold and Thompson, Helen: The Psychology of Early Growth, New York, 1938, The Macmillan Co.

Johnson, B. J.: Child Psychology, Springfield, Ill., and Baltimore, Md., 1932, Charles C. Thomas.

Kanner, Leo: Child Psychiatry, Springfield, Ill., 1935, Charles C. Thomas.

Myerson, Abraham: The Nervous Housewife, Boston, 1927, Little, Brown & Co.

Oliver, J. R.: Psychiatry and Mental Health, New York, 1932, Charles Scribner's Sons.

Sachs, Bernard: Keeping Your Child Normal, New York, 1936, Paul B. Hoeber, Inc.

Stiles, Percy G.: The Nervous System and Its Conservation, ed. 3, revised, Philadelphia, 1924, W. B. Saunders Company.

Taylor, W. S.: Readings in Abnormal Psychology and Mental Hygiene, New York, 1926, D. Appleton & Co.

Zachry, Caroline B.: Emotion and Conduct in Adolescence, New York, 1940, D. Appleton-Century Co.

Questions for Chapter XXIX

Mental Hygiene

1. Explain the meaning of "mental hygiene."
2. Is the term used in a broad or a narrow sense?
3. How did the mental hygiene movement demonstrate its breadth of outlook early in its career?
4. What are the fundamental aims of the mental hygiene movement?
5. Discuss child guidance.
6. What is an orthopsychiatrist?
7. What are some faulty elementary habits which children may form and which should be corrected?
8. Discuss adolescence and the necessity for application of mental hygiene methods at this time.
9. What are some abnormal personality traits which may emerge at the time of adolescence?
10. What can you do as a nurse to stimulate the interest of your community in mental hygiene?

malaria - Quartan - runs q 72 hrs - q 4 days,

GLOSSARY

Many of the terms used in psychiatric literature are not strictly technical, and a definition can usually be found in any good standard English dictionary. In the short list which follows are terms which have not been defined in the text and which may be frequently encountered in lectures and discussions. For a more complete and very practical lexicon, the reader is referred to the *Psychiatric Word Book* by Richard H. Hutchings, M.D., published by the State Hospitals Press, Utica, N. Y., under the auspices of the New York State Department of Mental Hygiene. A larger "Psychiatric Dictionary" and equally useful is one by Leland E. Hinsie and Jacob Shatzky, published in 1940 by the Oxford University Press of New York.

A

Abasia, unsteadiness in walking.

Abulia, absence or deficiency in will power.

Acrophobia, terror of being on high places.

Affect, emotion or mood and all the reactions arising with it.

Affective psychosis, a psychosis which is dominated by a sustained mood.

Agoraphobia, morbid fear when in wide open spaces.

Alienist, a physician testifying before a court on insanity.

Amentia, (1) feeblemindedness, oligophrenia; (2) acute hallucinatory confusional state associated with physical exhaustion; exhaustion delirium.

Anorexia, absence of appetite.

Aphonia, loss of voice.

Astasia, loss of ability to stand erect.

Astasia abasia, inability to stand erect or walk due to mental conflict.

Autism, living within one's self; introversion.

B

Behaviorism, a psychology which holds that only correct conclusions can be obtained from pure objective study of behavior.

322

Benign stupor, a stupor or apathy due to a mental disturbance as contrasted with a stupor or coma due to physical disease such as brain tumor or uremia. The term is usually applied to the depressed type of manic-depressive psychosis.

Bestiality, sexual connection with an animal.

Blocking, sudden obstruction of flow of thought due to the arousal of a painful thought or conflict.

C

Catalepsy, stupor with rigidity of the muscles seen in hysteria.

Cataplexy, sudden, short attack of complete loss of muscular tone, and voluntary muscular power; consciousness is retained.

Catathymic thinking, thinking which is determined by an emotion.

Catatonia, a stupor associated with muscular tension or cerea flexibilitas.

Cerea flexibilitas, waxlike flexibility of the muscles seen in catatonia: the limbs of the patient can be placed in any position and will remain there for varying lengths of time.

Circumstantiality, a type of speaking which reaches its goal only after relating many unnecessary details and incidents.

Claustrophobia, morbid fear when in enclosed or narrow spaces.

Clonus, hyperirritability of a reflex causing sustained oscillation of an extremity.

Cognition, awareness and understanding of objects through the functioning of one's senses; knowing.

Coitus interruptus, termination of coitus by withdrawal before completion of the act, usually done to avoid deposition of semen.

Coma, a profound stupor from which the patient is aroused with great difficulty.

Conation, a primary urge or instinctual striving.

Concept, a mental image.

Confabulation, the recital of imaginary experiences to cover a period of memory loss.

Conflict, a state of tension and painful consciousness due to the patient not being able to satisfy opposing urges.

Consciousness, clear awareness of self and the environment.

Constitutional, pertaining to inherited attributes.

Cortex, the outer layer of the cerebrum.

Cyclothymia, a term applied to mild recurrent mood swings of exhilaration and depression occurring in the syntonic personality.

D

Delusion, a false idea which cannot be corrected by adequate proof of its falsity.

Delusion of reference, false beliefs derived from casual incidents or remarks which are given an interpretation in reference to self.

Dementia, a deterioration of mental powers.

Depersonalization, a feeling of being someone else.

Dereistic, mental interests which are away from reality, daydreaming, phantasy.

Diathesis, an inherited or congenital tendency to develop a certain type of disease.

Dipsomania, periodic drinking of alcoholic beverages in response to some pathological mental state as depression.

Dissociation, a condition in which feeling, acting, and thinking are not in harmony.

Dual personality, a condition in which the patient leads two lives as if he were two different persons, neither personality being fully aware of the existence of the other.

Dynamic psychology, psychology which stresses the existence of mental forces which energetically demand expression.

Dysarthria, inability in pronunciation.

E

Echolalia, senseless repetition of words heard spoken by others.

Ecomania, domineering and haughty attitude toward people in the family circle and compliance and humility toward persons in authority.

Ego, that part of the personality which is conscious and in contact with reality through the sense organs. It constantly seeks to harmonize instinctual desires with the ethical and moral code of society.

Ego instincts, all instincts excluding sex; self-preservation and the herd instinct.

Empathy, the ability to understand another's emotions but not to ''feel with him.''

Encephalitis, inflammation of the brain.

Erotism, the affective element in the sexual impulse. Sexual excitement.

Euphoria, extraordinary feeling of well-being.

Exhibitionism, the display of the body or any of its parts to arouse sexual interest.

Extroversion, focusing of interests on the outside world.

F

Fabrication, relating imaginary events as true.

Free association, the spontaneous association of ideas which occurs when censorship is removed.

G

Globus hystericus, the sensation of having a ball in the throat; it is a hysterical spasm of the esophagus.

H

Hallucination, a sensory experience occurring in the absence of a sensory stimulus.

Hebetude, dullness, lethargy.

Hemiplegia, paralysis of one side of the body.

Heterosexuality, love of a person of the opposite sex.

Homosexuality, love of persons of the same sex.

Hyperprosexia, one idea dominating consciousness to the exclusion of others, seen in obsessional and compulsion neuroses.

Hyperthymia, increased emotional response to stimuli.

Hypertonus, heightened tension of a muscle.

Hypnosis, a sleeplike state induced by suggestion during which attention is focused on the operator.

Hypochondriasis, a condition in which there is excessive preoccupation with bodily organs. The subject thinks they are diseased.

I

Id, the unconscious part of the personality containing dynamic instinctive urges. It continually seeks gratification of its desires.

Idiopathic, term applied to diseases of unknown cause, such as idiopathic epilepsy.

Infantilism, applied to adults who are childish or immature mentally or physically.

Integration, bringing together components into a harmonious structure.

Introversion, focusing of interest on the internal world of self.

J

Jacksonian epilepsy, convulsive movements in limited groups of muscles, sometimes in a definite order; consciousness is usually not lost.

K

Kleptomania, morbid impulse to steal useless and petty things.

L

Labile, smooth flowing, flexible.

Lethargic, sleepy, somnolent, dull.

Libido, the energy contained in the sexual instinct. It includes not only sexual love, but also love for children, parents, friends and love of humanity in general.

Logorrhea, continuous excessive flow of speech, coherent but repetitious.

Lucid interval, a period during which there is a remission of symptoms in a psychosis.

M

Malingerer, a person who consciously feigns an illness or disability.

Megalomania, a condition in which there are delusions of great self-importance, power or wealth.

Menacme, the period in a woman's life when she is capable of bearing children; between puberty and the menopause.

Milieu, the environment, the people and objects with which the individual deals.

Misogamy, dislike of being married.

Misogyny, morbid dislike or hate of women.

Mnemic, having to do with memory.

Monoplegia, paralysis of one extremity.

Mysophobia, fear of dirt or contamination.

N

Narcissism, self-love. An early stage of psychosexual development when the love object is the individual himself.

Narcolepsy, a condition in which the individual is overcome by short irresistible periods of sleep.

Necrophobia, a morbid fear of dead bodies.

Negativism, a response which is opposite to that which is normal or called for in a given instance.

Neologism, a word which is coined by the individual and is meaningless to the hearer.

Neuron, the nerve cell and its processes, the fundamental unit of the nervous system.

Nihilistic delusion, a delusion that the world or universe has ended.

Nosophobia, unreasonable fear of illness, usually fear of a particular disease.

Nostalgia, homesickness.

Nudophobia, morbid fear of being unclothed.

Nyctophobia, exaggerated fear of darkness.

O

Ochlophobia, fear of being in crowds.

Ombrophobia, fear of threatening storms, rain, or dark clouds.

Onanism, masturbation.

Oral erotism, pleasurable sensation obtained from the mouth. First experience in suckling at the breast. Later modified and sublimated but still persisting as in kissing.

Orgasm, the peak of sexual pleasure, accompanied in the male by ejaculation.

Orthopsychiatry, the study of behavior disorders particularly in children and adolescents.

P

Palsy, paresis or paralysis of a muscle or group of muscles.

Parabulia, any abnormality of the will.

Paragraphia, writing wrong words or letters due to disease of the visual word center.

Paralexia, inability to understand written words or sentences.

Paresis, weakness of a muscle or group of muscles.

Parosmia, any disturbance in the sense of smell.

Pavor nocturnus, terror occurring during sleep; most often seen in children.

Perception, the act of becoming aware of a sensory stimulus.

Peripheral, away from the center, at the edge, close to the exterior, distal.

Perversion, substitution of another aim for the usual aim in any activity. Usually related to sexual activity when a component of sex or an earlier stage of sexual development is substituted for normal coitus.

Phlegmatic, a sluggish, nonexcitable temperament.

Phobia, an abnormal fear.

Photophobia, fear of light; inability of the eyes to endure light.

Preconscious, a subdivision of the mind holding ideas which are not conscious but which can readily be recalled to consciousness.

Presbyopia, farsightedness developing with advancing age.

Prison psychosis, a psychosis occurring in psychopaths awaiting trial or serving a sentence.

Psyche, the mind; the mental aspects of a person.

Psychiatry, the study and treatment of mental disease.

Psychodynamic, a term which refers to the interplay of mental forces in the individual's attempt to adjust to his environment.

Psychogenesis, the origin and development of mental phenomena.

Psycholepsy, a term referring to sudden changes in affect or mental tension.

Psychology, that branch of science which treats of mental functions.

Psychometry, the use of intelligence tests.

Psychosexual, pertaining to the mental components of the sexual instinct.

Psychrophobia, abnormal fear of cold.

Puerilism, childishness; applied to adults who have the mental or physical traits usually associated with childhood.

Pyknolepsy, a syndrome consisting of sudden, recurrent, momentary interruptions of consciousness usually in children. It is not true epilepsy.

Pyromania, an abnormal impulse to start fires.

Pyrophobia, abnormal fear of fire.

R

Rapport, a confidential relationship between physician and patient.

Regression, the return of the personality to some earlier, simpler stage of development, because of inability to properly function at an adult level.

Resistance, the mental force which tries to prevent repressed material from entering consciousness.

Rorschach test, a test which attempts to measure the affective components of personality.

S

Sadism, sexual pleasure obtained by inflicting pain on another person.

Schizo-, to split.

Scotophobia, morbid dread of darkness.

Sensorium, that mental capacity which makes the individual clearly aware of his immediate environment.

Sinistrality, lefthandedness.

Soma, the body, the physical aspect of man as distinguished from the psyche.

Somatic, bodily, having reference to the body or its organs.

Spasticity, a state of increased muscular tone resulting in stiffness and difficulty in moving.

Stereotypy, apparently senseless repetition of words or acts, seen in schizophrenia.

Subconscious, a portion of the mind not clearly conscious but which can be made conscious by exercising memory or through the association of ideas.

Suggestibility, referring to a person's susceptibility to having his ideas or actions changed by the influence of others.

Superego, that part of the personality which represses and judges the ego according to the moral and ethical codes of society. Analogous to conscience.

Symbol, anything which represents or stands for something else.

Syntonic, a type of personality in which thinking, feeling, and acting blend harmoniously.

Syphilophobia, abnormal fear of acquiring syphilis.

T

Topophobia, abnormal fear of some particular place.

Trance, a transient mental state in which consciousness is entirely or partially obliterated.

Transference, an extreme form of psychological rapport, an emotional tie of dependence between patient and physician based on identification.

Transvestitism, a sexual perversion in which pleasure of a sexual nature is obtained by dressing in the clothes of the opposite sex.

Twilight state, a state of partial clouding of consciousness in which evidently purposeful acts are committed with subsequent amnesia for them—seen in hysteria and epilepsy.

U

Unconscious, a portion of the mental apparatus attached to the id which contains repressed material. It is not accessible to consciousness but can be investigated by psychoanalysis.

V

Verbigeration, a stereotypy in which a word or phrase is continually repeated.

Volition, the will.

W

Word salad, voluble speech in which words and phrases have no logical connection or meaning.

X

Xenophobia, abnormal fear of strangers.

Z

Zones, erotic, regions such as the lips, breasts, genito-anal area, etc., stimulation of which causes erotic excitement.

Zoophobia, abnormal fear of animals; usually with reference to harmless domestic animals.

Zooscopic hallucinations, visual hallucinations of animals, most frequently seen in delirium tremens.

Types of Hydro-theropy
1. Continuous tub — 94° or 95° H_2O

Wet sheet Pack —
First Stage — Cooling Stage — Should last 8 to 20 min.
2nd Stage — Sedative "

INDEX

A

Accidents on mental wards, 85
Acromegaly, psychosis with, 167
Acute alcoholic psychoses, treatment of, 169
  chorea, psychoses with, 159
  depression, symptoms of, 106
  hallucinosis, alcoholic, 172
  mania, case illustrating, 100
    definition of, 98
    treatment of, 112
Addison's disease, 168
Adolescence, factor in mental disease, 53
  mental hygiene in, 319
Adrenal hormone in bromide poisoning, 183
Affective-reaction psychoses:
  involutional psychoses, 117-128
  manic-depressive psychoses, 92-116
Age factor in mental disease, 53
Alcohol:
  acute hallucinosis, 170
  acute reactions to, 170
  chronic reactions to, 170
  delirium tremens, 170
  effects of, 169
  factor in mental disease, 54
  general use of, 169
  pathological intoxication from, 170
Alcoholic dementia, 170
  deterioration, 170
    description of, 177
  hallucinosis, acute, case illustrating, 173
    description of, 172
  Korsakow's psychosis, 170
  paranoia, case illustrating, 170, 175-176
  psychoses, 169
    causes of, 169
    percentage of, 170
    treatment of, 173
    types of, 170
Alcoholism, chronic, commitment of, 177
  spinal function in, 174
  treatment of, 177

Alienist, 308
Alzheimer's disease, 213
Amaurotic family idiocy, 236
Amnesia, 255
Amphetamine sulphate in depression, 115
  encephalitis, 206
"Anatomy of Melancholy," by Burton, 21
Angiography, 69
Anxiety state, 248
  case illustrating, 249
  definition of, 247
  symptoms of, 248
Arsenical compounds in treatment of syphilis, 194
Arteriosclerosis, cerebral, mental symptoms in, 209-210
  treatment of, 211
Asthenic body type, 38, 58
Athletic body type, 39

B

Barbital intoxication, treatment of, 179
Barbituric acid intoxication, 183
Basal ganglia, 42
Beard and term "neurasthenia," 247
"Bedlam," 21
Beers, Clifford: "A Mind That Found Itself," 24
Behavior chart, reproduction of, 87
  terminology in, 88
Benzedrine sulphate (see Amphetamine)
Bethlem Hospital, 20
Binet-Simon intelligence test, Stanford Revision of, 229
  outline of, 230
Bini, L., 301
Birth palsy, cerebral, 236
Bismuth, in general paresis, 194
Bleuler, Eugen, 92
Brain cells, changes in Korsakow's psychoses, 175
Brain tumor, mental symptoms of, 202
  nursing care of, 204
  psychoses with, 202

331

Pinel, 21, 22
Pons and cerebellum, 40
Post-traumatic constitution in psychoneuroses, 197-198
Prefrontal lobotomy (*see* Psychosurgery)
Presenile dementia, 213
Privileged communications, 312
Projection, examples of, 47
Psychasthenia, 257
  case illustrating, 259
  phobias in, 259
  symptoms of, 258
Psychoanalysis, 264
Psychobiology, 52
Psychogenic factors, 59
Psychoneuroses, 245
  causes of, 246
  classification of, 247
  definition of, 245
  heredity in, 31
  nursing care of, 266
  treatment of, 262
Psychopathic personality, 239
  case illustrating, 242
  description of, 239
  prognosis in, 243
  sexual aberrations in, 241
  treatment of, 243
Psychosomatic medicine, 52
Psychosurgery, 127
  in involutional melancholia, 127
  in psychasthenia, 261
Psychotherapy, definition of, 262
Puerperal psychoses, 160
Pyknic body type, 38, 57

R

Rage, explanation of, 36
Rapport, 263
Rationalization, 46
Reaction type, paranoid, 152
  psychoses with endocrine disease, 163
  psychoses with somatic disease, 158
Recessive characters in heredity, 29
Recreational therapy, 286
Re-education, 264
Repression, 47
Restraint, 77
Roman civilization, 18, 19
Rorschach Test, 67
Royal touch, 19
Rush, Benjamin, 22

S

Sacred disease, 18
Sakel, Manfred, 25
  and insulin shock therapy, 289
Saul, King, 18
Schizoid personality, 129
Schizophrenia, affect in, 129
  catatonic type, 140
  definition of, 130
  etiology of, 130
  hebephrenic type, 136
  heredity in, 31
  ideas of persecution in, 131
  nursing care in, 147
  paranoid type, 145
  regression in, 138
  shock treatment of, 150
  simple, case illustrating, 132-134
  symptoms of, 131
  treatment in, 147
  types of, 132
Schizothymic body type, 38
Scotch douche, 279
Self-injury, precautions against, 83
Senile dementia, paranoid type, 216
  precipitating factors, 218
  treatment of, 217
  deterioration, 217
  psychoses, delirious and confused types, 216
  depressed and agitated types, 216
  nursing care of, 219
  paranoid type, 216
  presbyophrenic types, 217
  simple deterioration in, 215
  types of, 214
Sex, Freud on, 35
  heterosexual, 36
  homosexual, 35
  instinct of, 34
  narcissistic, 35
Shatzky, Jacob, 322
Shell shock, 256
Skull, trepanning of, 17
Shock therapy, in depression, 115
  in mental disease, 289
  insulin, 289-294
  metrazol, 294-301
Sitz bath, 271
Sleep, regulation of, 82
Sleeplessness (*see* Insomnia)
Spinal cord, 40
  fluid in general paresis, 191
  puncture in alcoholics, 174

Phobia :

Acarophobia — Fear of vermon, or itch
Agoraphobia — " " open spaces
Acrophobia — " " high places
Anthro — " " people
Astro — " " heavens, thunder & lightening
Auto — " " of solitude, or being alone
Bacterio — " " Bacteria or germs
Bato — " " high things falling.
Claustro — " " closed places —
Ergo — " " work
Erythro — " " Blushing
Lysso — " " rabies
Mono — " " being alone
Myso — " " filth or contamination
Necro — " " death or dead bodies
Neo — " " new things or unusual.
Nudo — " " unclothed —
Nycto — " " darkness
Noso " " of sickness
Ochlo — Fear of crowds —
Ombro — " " threatening storms, rain, or dark clouds —
Pano — " " everything or some vague evil.
Phobo — " " own fears —
Photo — " " sensitivity of light.
Psycho — " " insanity of self.
Psychro " " cold
Pyro " " fire
Scoto — " " abnormal or morbid fear of darkness —
Siderodromo — " " railroad travel.
Sito — " " eating.
Terato — " " monsters or of giving birth to monsters.
Topo — " " particular place.
Thanato — " " death.

"Inferiority Complex" Implies use of a real or assumed inferiority as a means of excuse, as a demand for special service or consideration. A frequent neurotic mechanism of escape.)

Inferiority feelings - may actually lead to the development of positive qualities and accomplishments. because individual may be aware of inadequacy, thus permitting compensatory endeavors. Indiv. may also be unaware of inferior feelings. whereas:

Inferiority complex — Inhibits progress. It is a final conclusion of hopelessness, whether it is limited to a certain area of activity or in the total social scene. The individual "knows" he or she is no good or cannot do something.

The most painful experience for any child or adult is the feeling that he is inferior to others.

The feeling of not belonging is the greatest hardship for any human being.!

Social interest, the feeling of belonging, is expressed by the desire and willingness to participate, to contribute, and to meet difficult situations without withdrawal.

19 - 20 17